ACID REFLUX AND GERD DIET COOKBOOK FOR BEGINNERS

Easy, Fast And Delicious Recipes for Healing and Relief From LPR. Overcome Heartburn and Maintain Healthy Gut.

Olivia Endwell

Copyright Statement:

Disclaimer:

Individual results may vary, and the success of any dietary or lifestyle change depends on various factors, including but not limited to individual commitment and adherence. Before making significant changes to your diet or lifestyle, consult with a qualified healthcare professional.

The views and opinions expressed in this book are those of the author and do not necessarily reflect the official policy or position of any other agency, organization, employer, or company.

TABLE OF CONTENTS

INTRODUCTION

In the rolling hills of Virginia, there lived a woman named Evelyn. She used to love the simple pleasures of life—like eating good food with friends—but that joy faded when she was diagnosed with acid reflux and GERD.

GERD stands for Gastroesophageal Reflux Disease, which is a condition where stomach acid flows back into the esophagus, causing discomfort and irritation. Acid reflux is similar but more temporary— it's when stomach acid occasionally flows back into the esophagus, leading to heartburn or a sour taste in the mouth.

Evelyn's nights were rough. She'd toss and turn, feeling a burning pain in her throat and chest. Eating became a struggle, as even the smallest bite could set off discomfort.

But Evelyn wasn't one to give up easily. She turned to her grandma's advice and decided to change her diet to help her body heal. In her kitchen, she experimented with different foods, learning which ones made her feel better and which ones made things worse.

Day by day, Evelyn's efforts paid off. She started feeling better, the pain lessening with each passing week. She discovered new favorite foods that didn't upset her stomach, like roasted veggies and whole grains.

As Evelyn's own journey progressed, she felt a pull to help others facing similar struggles. She became a listening ear and a source of comfort for those going through the same challenges she once did.

In the end, Evelyn's story wasn't just about her own healing. It was about finding strength in tough times, making small changes that lead to big improvements, and spreading kindness to others along the way. And through her experience, she shed light on what it means to live with GERD and acid reflux, inspiring others to seek help and make positive changes for their own well-being.

UNDERSTANDING ACID REFLUX AND GERD

What is Acid Reflux?

Acid reflux, also known as gastroesophageal reflux (GER), occurs when the acidic contents of the stomach flow back into the esophagus. The esophagus is the tube that carries food and liquids from the mouth to the stomach. Normally, a ring of muscle called the lower esophageal sphincter (LES) prevents the contents of the stomach from refluxing into the esophagus. However, when the LES becomes weakened or relaxes abnormally, stomach acid can escape into the esophagus, leading to symptoms such as heartburn, regurgitation, and chest pain.

Acid reflux often occurs after eating large meals, lying down immediately after eating, or consuming certain trigger foods and beverages such as spicy foods, citrus fruits, caffeine, alcohol, and carbonated drinks. While occasional acid reflux is common and usually harmless, frequent or severe episodes may indicate gastroesophageal reflux disease (GERD), a more chronic and serious condition.

What is GERD?

GERD, short for gastroesophageal reflux disease, is a chronic condition characterized by frequent and persistent acid reflux. Unlike occasional acid reflux, which may be triggered by specific foods or activities, GERD involves persistent symptoms that occur two or more times per week and can significantly impact a person's quality of life. In addition to heartburn and regurgitation, individuals with GERD may experience symptoms such as chest pain, difficulty swallowing (dysphagia), chronic cough, and hoarseness.

GERD is often the result of a malfunctioning lower esophageal sphincter (LES), which fails to close properly and allows stomach acid to flow back into the esophagus. Other contributing factors to GERD may include obesity, hiatal hernia (a condition in which part of the stomach protrudes into the chest cavity), pregnancy, smoking, and certain medications such as nonsteroidal anti-inflammatory drugs (NSAIDs) and calcium channel blockers.

Causes of Acid Reflux and GERD

Several factors can contribute to the development of acid reflux and GERD. One of the primary causes is a malfunctioning lower esophageal sphincter (LES), which fails to close properly and allows stomach acid to flow back into the esophagus. This can occur due to a variety of reasons, including obesity, pregnancy, hiatal hernia, and certain medications.

Obesity is a significant risk factor for both acid reflux and GERD. Excess weight can put pressure on the abdomen, causing the stomach contents to be pushed upward into the esophagus. Additionally, abdominal fat may affect the function of the LES, further increasing the likelihood of acid reflux.

Pregnancy can also contribute to the development of acid reflux and GERD. Hormonal changes during pregnancy can relax the LES, allowing stomach acid to reflux into the esophagus more easily. Furthermore, as the uterus expands, it can exert pressure on the stomach, further exacerbating acid reflux symptoms.

Hiatal hernia is another common cause of acid reflux and GERD. This condition occurs when a portion of the stomach protrudes through the diaphragm and into the chest cavity, disrupting the normal function of the LES. As a result, stomach acid may reflux into the esophagus, leading to symptoms of GERD.

Certain medications can also increase the risk of acid reflux and GERD. Nonsteroidal anti-inflammatory drugs (NSAIDs) such as ibuprofen and aspirin can irritate the esophagus and weaken the LES, making reflux more likely. Similarly, calcium channel blockers, used to treat conditions such as high blood pressure, can relax the LES and contribute to GERD symptoms.

In addition to these factors, smoking, excessive alcohol consumption, and certain dietary habits (such as consuming spicy or fatty foods) can also increase the risk of acid reflux and GERD. By understanding the potential causes of these conditions, individuals can take steps to reduce their risk and manage their symptoms effectively.

Symptoms of Acid Reflux and GERD

Acid reflux and GERD can cause a variety of symptoms, ranging from mild to severe. Common symptoms of acid reflux include heartburn, which is characterized by a burning sensation in the chest that may worsen after eating or lying down. Regurgitation, or the sensation of stomach contents coming back up into the throat or mouth, is another hallmark symptom of acid reflux.

In addition to heartburn and regurgitation, individuals with acid reflux may experience other symptoms such as chest pain, difficulty swallowing (dysphagia), and a sour or bitter taste in the mouth. Chronic cough, hoarseness, and throat irritation are also common symptoms, particularly if stomach acid reaches the throat and larynx.

GERD, being a more chronic and severe form of acid reflux, often involves persistent and frequent symptoms that significantly impact a person's quality of life. In addition to the symptoms mentioned above, individuals with GERD may experience chest pain that mimics a heart attack, difficulty swallowing (especially with solid foods), and a persistent sore throat or hoarseness.

It's important to note that not everyone with acid reflux or GERD will experience all of these symptoms, and the severity of symptoms can vary from person to person. Some individuals may only experience occasional heartburn or regurgitation, while others may have more frequent and severe symptoms that require medical intervention. By recognizing the common symptoms of acid reflux and GERD, individuals can seek appropriate treatment and management strategies to improve their quality of life.

Complications of Untreated Acid Reflux and GERD

Untreated acid reflux and GERD can lead to a variety of complications, ranging from mild to severe. One of the most common complications is esophagitis, which is inflammation or irritation of the esophagus due to prolonged exposure to stomach acid. Esophagitis can cause symptoms such as difficulty swallowing (dysphagia), chest pain, and bleeding.

Chronic acid reflux and GERD can also increase the risk of developing Barrett's esophagus, a condition characterized by changes in the cells lining the lower esophagus. While Barrett's esophagus itself may not cause symptoms, it is considered a precancerous condition and can increase the risk of developing esophageal cancer.

In addition to Barrett's esophagus, untreated acid reflux and GERD can lead to other complications such as esophageal strictures (narrowing of the esophagus due to scarring), respiratory problems (such as asthma or aspiration pneumonia), and dental erosions (due to exposure to stomach acid). Chronic cough, hoarseness, and laryngitis may also occur as a result of acid reflux reaching the throat and larynx.

Furthermore, untreated GERD can significantly impact a person's quality of life, leading to sleep disturbances, reduced productivity, and impaired social functioning. Chronic pain, discomfort, and anxiety related to acid reflux symptoms can also contribute to mental health issues such as depression and anxiety.

Overall, the complications of untreated acid reflux and GERD underscore the importance of seeking appropriate treatment and management strategies to prevent long-term damage to the esophagus and improve overall quality of life. By addressing symptoms early and implementing lifestyle changes and medical interventions as needed, individuals can reduce their risk of complications and enjoy better health outcomes in the long term.

THE ACID REFLUX AND GERD DIET: BASICS

Importance of Diet in Managing Acid Reflux and GERD

Diet plays a crucial role in managing acid reflux and gastroesophageal reflux disease (GERD). While medications can help alleviate symptoms, dietary modifications are often recommended as a first-line approach to reduce the frequency and severity of reflux episodes. A well-planned diet can help minimize the amount of stomach acid that flows back into the esophagus, thereby reducing irritation and discomfort.

One of the primary goals of a GERD-friendly diet is to avoid foods and beverages that can trigger reflux symptoms. Certain foods, such as spicy foods, citrus fruits, tomatoes, chocolate, caffeine, and alcohol, are known to relax the lower esophageal sphincter (LES) or increase stomach acid production, making reflux more likely. By identifying and eliminating these trigger foods from the diet, individuals with acid reflux and GERD can reduce their risk of experiencing uncomfortable symptoms.

In addition to avoiding trigger foods, incorporating foods that are less likely to cause reflux can also help manage symptoms. These include non-citrus fruits, vegetables, whole grains, lean proteins, and low-fat dairy products. These foods are generally easier to digest and less likely to irritate the esophagus, making them suitable choices for individuals with acid reflux and GERD.

Furthermore, practicing portion control and meal timing is essential for managing acid reflux and GERD symptoms. Eating smaller, more frequent meals throughout the day can help prevent overeating and reduce pressure on the stomach, which can contribute to reflux. It's also important to avoid lying down immediately after eating, as this can increase the risk of acid reflux. Instead, waiting at least two to three hours before lying down can help ensure that food is properly digested before bedtime.

Overall, adopting a GERD-friendly diet can provide significant relief from symptoms and improve overall quality of life for individuals with acid reflux and GERD. By making mindful choices about the foods they eat and how they consume them, individuals can take control of their health and effectively manage their condition.

Foods to Avoid

When it comes to managing acid reflux and GERD, certain foods and beverages should be avoided or limited to reduce the risk of triggering reflux symptoms. These include:

1. Spicy Foods: Spicy foods such as chili peppers, hot sauces, and curry can irritate the esophagus and relax the lower esophageal sphincter (LES), making reflux more likely.

2. Citrus Fruits: Citrus fruits like oranges, lemons, grapefruits, and limes are highly acidic and can exacerbate acid reflux symptoms.

3. Tomatoes: Tomatoes and tomato-based products, such as tomato sauce and ketchup, are acidic and can increase stomach acid production, leading to reflux.

4. Chocolate: Chocolate contains caffeine and theobromine, both of which can relax the LES and stimulate stomach acid production, making reflux more likely.

5. Caffeine: Caffeinated beverages like coffee, tea, and soda can relax the LES and increase stomach acid production, leading to reflux symptoms.

6. Alcohol: Alcoholic beverages can irritate the esophagus and relax the LES, making reflux more likely. Red wine, in particular, is known to trigger reflux symptoms in some individuals.

7. Fatty Foods: High-fat foods like fried foods, fatty meats, and full-fat dairy products can delay stomach emptying and increase pressure on the LES, leading to reflux.

8. Carbonated Beverages: Carbonated beverages like soda and sparkling water can distend the stomach and increase pressure on the LES, making reflux more likely.

By avoiding or limiting these trigger foods and beverages, individuals with acid reflux and GERD can reduce the frequency and severity of reflux symptoms and improve their overall quality of life.

Foods to Include

In addition to avoiding trigger foods, incorporating GERD-friendly foods into the diet can help manage acid reflux and GERD symptoms. These include:

1. Non-Citrus Fruits: Non-citrus fruits such as bananas, apples, pears, and melons are lower in acidity and less likely to trigger reflux symptoms.

2. Vegetables: Most vegetables are well-tolerated by individuals with acid reflux and GERD. Leafy greens, broccoli, cauliflower, carrots, and potatoes are excellent choices.

3. Whole Grains: Whole grains such as oats, brown rice, quinoa, and barley are rich in fiber and less likely to cause reflux symptoms compared to refined grains.

4. Lean Proteins: Lean proteins like skinless poultry, fish, tofu, and legumes are easier to digest and less likely to trigger reflux compared to fatty meats.

5. Low-Fat Dairy Products: Low-fat dairy products like skim milk, yogurt, and cheese can be included in moderation as they are less likely to cause reflux compared to full-fat dairy products.

6. Herbs and Spices: While spicy foods should be avoided, mild herbs and spices like ginger, turmeric, and parsley can add flavor to dishes without triggering reflux.

7. Non-Caffeinated Beverages: Non-caffeinated beverages like water, herbal tea, and decaffeinated coffee can be consumed freely and are less likely to cause reflux symptoms.

8. Healthy Fats: Healthy fats such as olive oil, avocado, nuts, and seeds can be included in moderation and are less likely to trigger reflux compared to fried foods and fatty meats.

By including these GERD-friendly foods in their diet, individuals can enjoy a wide variety of flavorful and nutritious meals while minimizing the risk of experiencing uncomfortable reflux symptoms.

Portion Control and Meal Timing

Portion control and meal timing are important aspects of managing acid reflux and GERD symptoms. Eating large meals can put pressure on the stomach and increase the likelihood of reflux. To prevent overeating, individuals should aim to consume smaller, more frequent meals throughout the day. This can help reduce pressure on the stomach and prevent reflux episodes.

In addition to portion control, meal timing is also important for managing reflux symptoms. Eating meals too close to bedtime can increase the risk of reflux, as lying down shortly after eating can allow stomach acid to flow back into the esophagus more easily. To minimize the risk of nighttime reflux, individuals should avoid eating large meals or heavy snacks within two to three hours of bedtime.

Furthermore, it's important to pay attention to how meals are prepared and consumed. Eating slowly and chewing food thoroughly can aid digestion and reduce the risk of reflux. Avoiding tight clothing and maintaining an upright posture while eating can also help prevent reflux symptoms.

Overall, practicing portion control, mindful eating, and proper meal timing can help individuals with acid reflux and GERD manage their symptoms effectively and improve their overall quality of life.

Lifestyle Changes for Managing Acid Reflux and GERD

In addition to dietary modifications, certain lifestyle changes can help manage acid reflux and GERD symptoms and reduce the frequency and severity of reflux episodes. These include:

1. Weight Management: Maintaining a healthy weight is important for managing acid reflux and GERD, as excess weight can put pressure on the abdomen and increase the risk of reflux. Losing weight through diet and exercise can help alleviate reflux symptoms and improve overall health.

2. Smoking Cessation: Smoking can weaken the lower esophageal sphincter (LES) and increase stomach acid production, making reflux more likely. Quitting smoking can help reduce reflux symptoms and improve esophageal health.

3. Elevating the Head of the Bed: Elevating the head of the bed by six to eight inches can help prevent nighttime reflux by gravity. This allows gravity to keep stomach acid in the stomach and prevent it from flowing back into the esophagus while sleeping.

4. Avoiding Tight Clothing: Wearing tight clothing, especially around the abdomen, can put pressure on the stomach and increase the risk of reflux. Opting for loose-fitting clothing can help reduce pressure on the abdomen and alleviate reflux symptoms.

5. Stress Management: Stress can exacerbate acid reflux and GERD symptoms by increasing stomach acid production and affecting digestion. Practicing stress-reducing techniques such as deep breathing, meditation, yoga, and exercise can help alleviate reflux symptoms and improve overall well-being.

6. Sleeping Position: Sleeping on the left side can help prevent nighttime reflux by keeping the stomach below the esophagus. This can help prevent stomach acid from flowing back into the esophagus while sleeping and reduce the risk of reflux symptoms.

7. Avoiding Trigger Activities: Certain activities, such as bending over, lifting heavy objects, and vigorous exercise, can increase intra-abdominal pressure and trigger reflux. Avoiding

these activities or taking breaks between meals and exercise can help reduce reflux symptoms.

By implementing these lifestyle changes in conjunction with dietary modifications, individuals with acid reflux and GERD can effectively manage their symptoms and improve their overall quality of life. Taking a holistic approach to treatment that addresses both dietary and lifestyle factors can help individuals achieve long-term relief from reflux symptoms and maintain optimal digestive health.

BREAKFAST RECIPES

1. Oatmeal with Banana and Almond Butter

Prep Time: 5 minutes

Cooking Time: 10 minutes

Serving Size: 1

Ingredients:

- 1/2 cup rolled oats

- 1 cup water or almond milk

- 1 ripe banana, sliced

- 1 tablespoon almond butter

- Optional: honey or maple syrup for sweetness (avoid if sensitive to sweeteners)

Instructions:

1. In a small saucepan, bring water or almond milk to a boil.

2. Stir in rolled oats and reduce heat to low. Cook for 5-7 minutes, stirring occasionally, until oats are soft and creamy.

3. Transfer oatmeal to a bowl and top with sliced banana and almond butter.

4. Drizzle with honey or maple syrup if desired.

5. Serve warm and enjoy!

Nutritional Information (per serving):

- Calories: 350

- Protein: 9g

- Carbohydrates: 55g

- Fat: 11g

- Fiber: 8g

2. Greek Yogurt Parfait

Prep Time: 5 minutes

Serving Size: 1

Ingredients:

- 1/2 cup plain Greek yogurt

- 1/4 cup granola (choose low-fat, low-sugar options)

- 1/2 cup mixed berries (such as strawberries, blueberries, raspberries)

- 1 tablespoon honey (optional)

Instructions:

1. In a serving glass or bowl, layer plain Greek yogurt, granola, and mixed berries.

2. Repeat layers until ingredients are used up.

3. Drizzle with honey if desired.

4. Serve immediately and enjoy!

Nutritional Information (per serving):

- Calories: 250

- Protein: 15g

- Carbohydrates: 35g

- Fat: 5g

- Fiber: 6g

3. Scrambled Tofu with Spinach and Tomatoes

Prep Time: 10 minutes

Cooking Time: 10 minutes

Serving Size: 2

Ingredients:

- 1/2 block firm tofu, crumbled

- 1 cup fresh spinach leaves

- 1/2 cup cherry tomatoes, halved

- 1/4 teaspoon turmeric powder

- Salt and pepper to taste

- 1 tablespoon olive oil

Instructions:

1. Heat olive oil in a non-stick skillet over medium heat.

2. Add crumbled tofu to the skillet and cook for 2-3 minutes, stirring occasionally.

3. Add spinach leaves and cherry tomatoes to the skillet. Cook for another 3-4 minutes until vegetables are wilted and tofu is heated through.

4. Season with turmeric powder, salt, and pepper to taste. Stir well to combine.

5. Remove from heat and serve hot.

Nutritional Information (per serving):

- Calories: 180

- Protein: 12g

- Carbohydrates: 7g

- Fat: 12g

- Fiber: 3g

4. Banana Pancakes

Prep Time: 10 minutes

Cooking Time: 10 minutes

Serving Size: 2-3 pancakes

Ingredients:

- 1 ripe banana, mashed
- 2 eggs
- 1/4 teaspoon vanilla extract
- 1/4 teaspoon cinnamon
- Cooking spray or oil for greasing

Instructions:

1. In a mixing bowl, combine mashed banana, eggs, vanilla extract, and cinnamon. Mix until well combined.

2. Heat a non-stick skillet or griddle over medium heat and lightly grease with cooking spray or oil.

3. Pour about 1/4 cup of the pancake batter onto the skillet to form each pancake.

4. Cook for 2-3 minutes until bubbles form on the surface, then flip and cook for another 1-2 minutes until golden brown.

5. Repeat with remaining batter.

6. Serve warm with toppings of your choice, such as fresh fruit, Greek yogurt, or a drizzle of honey.

Nutritional Information (per serving, 2 pancakes):

- Calories: 150

- Protein: 7g

- Carbohydrates: 18g

- Fat: 6g

- Fiber: 2g

5. Avocado Toast with Poached Egg

Prep Time: 10 minutes

Cooking Time: 5 minutes

Serving Size: 1

Ingredients:

- 1 slice whole grain bread

- 1/2 ripe avocado, mashed

- 1 large egg

- Salt and pepper to taste

- Optional toppings: cherry tomatoes, sliced cucumber, microgreens

Instructions:

1. Toast the whole grain bread until golden brown.

2. Spread mashed avocado evenly over the toast.

3. Fill a small saucepan with water and bring to a gentle simmer.

4. Crack the egg into a small bowl, then gently slide it into the simmering water. Poach for 3-4 minutes until the whites are set but the yolk is still runny.

5. Using a slotted spoon, carefully remove the poached egg from the water and place it on top of the avocado toast.

6. Season with salt and pepper to taste.

7. Garnish with optional toppings if desired.

8. Serve immediately and enjoy!

Nutritional Information (per serving):

- Calories: 300

- Protein: 15g

- Carbohydrates: 20g

- Fat: 18g

- Fiber: 6g

6. Quinoa Breakfast Bowl

Prep Time: 5 minutes

Cooking Time: 15 minutes

Serving Size: 1

Ingredients:

- 1/2 cup cooked quinoa

- 1/4 cup unsweetened almond milk

- 1 tablespoon almond butter

- 1 tablespoon honey (optional)

- 1/4 cup mixed berries (such as strawberries, blueberries, raspberries)

- 1 tablespoon sliced almonds

- 1 teaspoon chia seeds

Instructions:

1. In a small saucepan, warm cooked quinoa with almond milk over medium heat until heated through.

2. Stir in almond butter and honey until well combined.

3. Transfer quinoa mixture to a serving bowl.

4. Top with mixed berries, sliced almonds, and chia seeds.

5. Serve warm and enjoy!

Nutritional Information (per serving):

- Calories: 350

- Protein: 10g

- Carbohydrates: 45g

- Fat: 15g

- Fiber: 7g

7. Apple Cinnamon Overnight Oats

Prep Time: 5 minutes (plus overnight soaking)

Serving Size: 1

Ingredients:

- 1/2 cup rolled oats

- 1/2 cup unsweetened almond milk

- 1/2 medium apple, grated

- 1/2 teaspoon cinnamon

- 1 tablespoon chopped walnuts

- Optional: honey or maple syrup for sweetness (avoid if sensitive to sweeteners)

Instructions:

1. In a mason jar or container, combine rolled oats, almond milk, grated apple, cinnamon, and chopped walnuts.

2. Stir well to combine all ingredients.

3. Cover the jar/container and refrigerate overnight, or for at least 4 hours.

4. In the morning, give the oats a good stir and add a drizzle of honey or maple syrup if desired.

5. Serve cold and enjoy!

Nutritional Information (per serving):

- Calories: 300

- Protein: 9g

- Carbohydrates: 45g

- Fat: 10g

- Fiber: 7g

8. Spinach and Feta Egg Muffins

Prep Time: 10 minutes

Cooking Time: 20 minutes

Serving Size: 2 muffins

Ingredients:

- 4 large eggs

- 1/4 cup unsweetened almond milk

- 1 cup fresh spinach leaves, chopped

- 1/4 cup crumbled feta cheese

- Salt and pepper to taste

- Cooking spray or oil for greasing

Instructions:

1. Preheat the oven to 350°F (175°C). Grease a muffin tin with cooking spray or oil.

2. In a mixing bowl, whisk together eggs and almond milk until well combined.

3. Stir in chopped spinach and crumbled feta cheese. Season with salt and pepper to taste.

4. Divide the egg mixture evenly among the muffin cups.

5. Bake for 20-25 minutes until the egg muffins are set and lightly golden brown on top.

6. Remove from the oven and allow to cool slightly before serving.

7. Serve warm or refrigerate for later use.

Nutritional Information (per serving, 2 muffins):

- Calories: 200

- Protein: 14g

- Carbohydrates: 3g

- Fat: 15g

- Fiber: 1g

9. Berry Smoothie Bowl

Prep Time: 5 minutes

Serving Size: 1

Ingredients:

- 1/2 cup frozen mixed berries (such as strawberries, blueberries, raspberries)

- 1/2 ripe banana

- 1/2 cup unsweetened almond milk

- 1 tablespoon chia seeds

- Toppings: sliced almonds, shredded coconut, fresh berries

Instructions:

1. In a blender, combine frozen mixed berries, banana, almond milk, and chia seeds.

2. Blend until smooth and creamy, adding more almond milk if needed to reach desired consistency.

3. Pour the smoothie into a serving bowl.

4. Top with sliced almonds, shredded coconut, and fresh berries.

5. Serve immediately and enjoy!

Nutritional Information (per serving):

- Calories: 250

- Protein: 6g

- Carbohydrates: 30g

- Fat: 12g

- Fiber: 10g

10. Veggie Breakfast Burrito

Prep Time: 10 minutes

Cooking Time: 10 minutes

Serving Size: 1

Ingredients:

- 1 whole grain tortilla

- 2 large eggs, scrambled

- 1/4 cup black beans, drained and rinsed

- 1/4 cup diced bell peppers

- 2 tablespoons diced onions

- 2 tablespoons shredded low-fat cheese

- Salsa and avocado for topping (optional)

Instructions:

1. In a non-stick skillet, scramble the eggs over medium heat until cooked through.

2. Warm the tortilla in the skillet or microwave until soft and pliable.

3. Spread the scrambled eggs in the center of the tortilla.

4. Top with black beans, diced bell peppers, onions, and shredded cheese.

5. Roll up the tortilla into a burrito.

6. If desired, serve with salsa and sliced avocado on top.

7. Serve warm and enjoy!

Nutritional Information (per serving):

- Calories: 350

- Protein: 22g

- Carbohydrates: 30g

- Fat: 15g

- Fiber: 7g

11. Sweet Potato Hash

Prep Time: 15 minutes

Cooking Time: 20 minutes

Serving Size: 2

Ingredients:

- 2 medium sweet potatoes, peeled and diced

- 1/2 onion, diced

- 1 bell pepper, diced

- 2 cloves garlic, minced

- 2 tablespoons olive oil

- 1 teaspoon paprika

- Salt and pepper to taste

- 2 eggs (optional, for topping)

Instructions:

1. Heat olive oil in a large skillet over medium heat.

2. Add diced sweet potatoes to the skillet and cook for 10-12 minutes, stirring occasionally, until tender and lightly browned.

3. Add diced onion, bell pepper, and minced garlic to the skillet. Cook for another 5-7 minutes until vegetables are softened.

4. Season with paprika, salt, and pepper to taste. Stir well to combine.

5. If desired, fry or poach eggs separately in another skillet.

6. Divide the sweet potato hash onto plates and top each serving with a fried or poached egg.

7. Serve hot and enjoy!

Nutritional Information (per serving):

- Calories: 300

- Protein: 8g

- Carbohydrates: 35g

- Fat: 15g

- Fiber: 6g

12. Cottage Cheese and Fruit Bowl

Prep Time: 5 minutes

Serving Size: 1

Ingredients:

- 1/2 cup low-fat cottage cheese

- 1/2 cup mixed berries (such as strawberries, blueberries, raspberries)

- 1 tablespoon chopped nuts (such as almonds, walnuts, or pecans)

- Optional: honey or maple syrup for sweetness (avoid if sensitive to sweeteners)

Instructions:

1. In a serving bowl, spoon low-fat cottage cheese.

2. Top with mixed berries and chopped nuts.

3. Drizzle with honey or maple syrup if desired.

4. Serve immediately and enjoy!

Nutritional Information (per serving):

- Calories: 200

- Protein: 15g

- Carbohydrates: 15g

- Fat: 10g

- Fiber: 5g

13. Chia Seed Pudding

Prep Time: 5 minutes (plus chilling time)
Serving Size: 1

Ingredients:

- 2 tablespoons chia seeds

- 1/2 cup unsweetened almond milk

- 1/4 teaspoon vanilla extract

- Optional toppings: sliced bananas, berries, shredded coconut

Instructions:

1. In a mason jar or container, combine chia seeds, almond milk, and vanilla extract.

2. Stir well to combine all ingredients.

3. Cover the jar/container and refrigerate for at least 2 hours, or overnight, until the chia seeds have absorbed the liquid and the mixture has thickened.

4. Stir the chia seed pudding again before serving.

5. Top with sliced bananas, berries, and shredded coconut if desired.

6. Serve chilled and enjoy!

Nutritional Information (per serving):

- Calories: 150

- Protein: 5g

- Carbohydrates: 15g

- Fat: 8g

- Fiber: 8g

14. Spinach and Mushroom Frittata

Prep Time: 10 minutes

Cooking Time: 20 minutes

Serving Size: 4

Ingredients:

- 6 large eggs

- 1/4 cup unsweetened almond milk

- 1 cup fresh spinach leaves, chopped

- 1/2 cup sliced mushrooms

- 1/4 cup diced onions

- 1/4 cup shredded low-fat cheese

- Salt and pepper to taste

- Cooking spray or oil for greasing

Instructions:

1. Preheat the oven to 350°F (175°C).

2. In a mixing bowl, whisk together eggs and almond milk until well combined.

3. Stir in chopped spinach, sliced mushrooms, diced onions, and shredded cheese. Season with salt and pepper to taste.

4. Grease a 9-inch pie dish with cooking spray or oil.

5. Pour the egg mixture into the pie dish.

6. Bake for 20-25 minutes until the frittata is set and lightly golden brown on top.

7. Remove from the oven and allow to cool slightly before slicing.

8. Serve warm or refrigerate for later use.

Nutritional Information (per serving):

- Calories: 150

- Protein: 12g

- Carbohydrates: 5g

- Fat: 8g

- Fiber: 1g

15. Almond Butter and Banana Smoothie

Prep Time: 5 minutes

Serving Size: 1

Ingredients:

- 1 ripe banana

- 1 tablespoon almond butter

- 1/2 cup unsweetened almond milk

- 1/2 cup ice cubes

- Optional: honey or maple syrup for sweetness (avoid if sensitive to sweeteners)

Instructions:

1. In a blender, combine ripe banana, almond butter, almond milk, and ice cubes.

2. Blend until smooth and creamy, adding more almond milk if needed to reach desired consistency.

3. Add a drizzle of honey or maple syrup if desired for sweetness.

4. Serve cold and enjoy!

Nutritional Information (per serving):

- Calories: 250

- Protein: 5g

- Carbohydrates: 30g

- Fat: 12g

- Fiber: 6g

16. Veggie Breakfast Wrap

Prep Time: 10 minutes
Cooking Time: 10 minutes
Serving Size: 1

Ingredients:

- 1 whole grain tortilla

- 2 large eggs, scrambled

- 1/4 cup diced bell peppers

- 1/4 cup diced onions

- 1/4 cup diced tomatoes

- 1/4 cup fresh spinach leaves

- 2 tablespoons shredded low-fat cheese

- Salt and pepper to taste

- Cooking spray or oil for greasing

Instructions:

1. In a non-stick skillet, scramble the eggs over medium heat until cooked through.

2. Warm the tortilla in the skillet or microwave until soft and pliable.

3. Spread the scrambled eggs in the center of the tortilla.

4. Top with diced bell peppers, onions, tomatoes, spinach leaves, and shredded cheese.

5. Season with salt and pepper to taste.

6. Roll up the tortilla into a wrap.

7. Serve warm and enjoy!

Nutritional Information (per serving):

- Calories: 300

- Protein: 18g

- Carbohydrates: 25g

- Fat: 12g

- Fiber: 6g

17. Blueberry Almond Chia Pudding

Prep Time: 5 minutes (plus chilling time)

Serving Size: 1

Ingredients:

- 2 tablespoons chia seeds

- 1/2 cup unsweetened almond milk

- 1/4 teaspoon almond extract

- 1/4 cup fresh blueberries

- 1 tablespoon sliced almonds

- Optional: honey or maple syrup for sweetness (avoid if sensitive to sweeteners)

Instructions:

1. In a mason jar or container, combine chia seeds, almond milk, and almond extract.

2. Stir well to combine all ingredients.

3. Gently fold in fresh blueberries.

4. Cover the jar/container and refrigerate for at least 2 hours, or overnight, until the chia seeds have absorbed the liquid and the mixture has thickened.

5. Stir the chia pudding again before serving.

6. Top with sliced almonds and a drizzle of honey or maple syrup if desired.

7. Serve chilled and enjoy!

Nutritional Information (per serving):

- Calories: 200

- Protein: 6g

- Carbohydrates: 20g

- Fat: 10g

- Fiber: 10g

18. Turkey and Veggie Breakfast Skillet

Prep Time: 10 minutes

Cooking Time: 15 minutes

Serving Size: 2

Ingredients:

- 4 large eggs

- 4 ounces lean turkey sausage, diced

- 1/2 bell pepper, diced

- 1/2 onion, diced

- 1 cup baby spinach leaves

- Salt and pepper to taste

- Cooking spray or oil for greasing

Instructions:

1. In a large skillet, cook diced turkey sausage over medium heat until browned and cooked through.

2. Add diced bell pepper and onion to the skillet. Cook for 3-4 minutes until softened.

3. Add baby spinach leaves to the skillet and cook for another 1-2 minutes until wilted.

4. Crack the eggs directly into the skillet over the sausage and vegetables.

5. Season with salt and pepper to taste.

6. Cook until the eggs are set to your desired level of doneness.

7. Divide the skillet mixture onto plates and serve hot.

Nutritional Information (per serving):

- Calories: 250

- Protein: 20g

- Carbohydrates: 10g

- Fat: 14g

- Fiber: 3g

19. Peanut Butter Banana Overnight Oats

Prep Time: 5 minutes (plus overnight soaking)

Serving Size: 1

Ingredients:

- 1/2 cup rolled oats

- 1/2 cup unsweetened almond milk

- 1 tablespoon peanut butter

- 1/2 ripe banana, sliced

- Optional: honey or maple syrup for sweetness (avoid if sensitive to sweeteners)

Instructions:

1. In a mason jar or container, combine rolled oats, almond milk, and peanut butter.

2. Stir well to combine all ingredients.

3. Gently fold in sliced banana.

4. Cover the jar/container and refrigerate overnight, or for at least 4 hours, until the oats have absorbed the liquid and the mixture has thickened.

5. Stir the oats again before serving.

6. Add a drizzle of honey or maple syrup if desired for sweetness.

7. Serve cold and enjoy!

Nutritional Information (per serving):

- Calories: 350

- Protein: 12g

- Carbohydrates: 45g

- Fat: 15g

- Fiber: 8g

20. Veggie Breakfast Casserole

Prep Time: 15 minutes

Cooking Time: 30 minutes

Serving Size: 6

Ingredients:

- 8 large eggs

- 1/2 cup unsweetened almond milk

- 1/2 cup diced bell peppers

- 1/2 cup diced onions

- 1 cup baby spinach leaves

- 1 cup diced tomatoes

- 1/2 cup shredded low-fat cheese

- Salt and pepper to taste

- Cooking spray or oil for greasing

Instructions:

1. Preheat the oven to 350°F (175°C). Grease a 9x13-inch baking dish with cooking spray or oil.

2. In a large mixing bowl, whisk together eggs and almond milk until well combined.

3. Stir in diced bell peppers, onions, spinach leaves, tomatoes, and shredded cheese. Season with salt and pepper to taste.

4. Pour the egg mixture into the prepared baking dish.

5. Bake for 25-30 minutes until the casserole is set and lightly golden brown on top.

6. Remove from the oven and allow to cool slightly before slicing.

7. Serve warm or refrigerate for later use.

Nutritional Information (per serving):

- Calories: 200

- Protein: 14g

- Carbohydrates: 10g

- Fat: 10g

- Fiber: 3g

LUNCH RECIPES

1. Grilled Chicken and Veggie Salad

Prep Time: 15 minutes

Cooking Time: 15 minutes

Serving Size: 2

Ingredients:

- 2 boneless, skinless chicken breasts
- 4 cups mixed salad greens
- 1 cup cherry tomatoes, halved
- 1/2 cucumber, sliced
- 1/4 red onion, thinly sliced
- 2 tablespoons olive oil
- 2 tablespoons balsamic vinegar
- Salt and pepper to taste

Instructions:

1. Preheat grill to medium-high heat.
2. Season chicken breasts with salt and pepper.
3. Grill chicken for 6-7 minutes per side until cooked through and no longer pink in the center.

4. In a large bowl, toss together mixed salad greens, cherry tomatoes, cucumber, and red onion.

5. In a small bowl, whisk together olive oil and balsamic vinegar to make the dressing.

6. Slice grilled chicken and place on top of the salad.

7. Drizzle salad with dressing.

8. Serve immediately and enjoy!

Nutritional Information (per serving):

- Calories: 300

- Protein: 25g

- Carbohydrates: 12g

- Fat: 15g

- Fiber: 4g

2. Turkey and Avocado Wrap

Prep Time: 10 minutes

Serving Size: 1

Ingredients:

- 1 whole grain tortilla

- 2 slices roasted turkey breast

- 1/4 avocado, sliced

- 1/4 cup mixed greens

- 1 tablespoon Greek yogurt

- 1 teaspoon Dijon mustard

Instructions:

1. Lay the whole grain tortilla flat on a clean surface.

2. Spread Greek yogurt and Dijon mustard over the tortilla.

3. Layer slices of roasted turkey breast, avocado, and mixed greens on top.

4. Roll up the tortilla tightly into a wrap.

5. Slice in half if desired and serve.

Nutritional Information (per serving):

- Calories: 250

- Protein: 20g

- Carbohydrates: 20g

- Fat: 10g

- Fiber: 6g

3. Salmon and Quinoa Salad

Prep Time: 20 minutes

Cooking Time: 15 minutes

Serving Size: 2

Ingredients:

- 2 salmon fillets

- 1 cup cooked quinoa

- 2 cups mixed salad greens

- 1/2 cup diced cucumber

- 1/2 cup cherry tomatoes, halved

- 2 tablespoons olive oil

- 1 tablespoon lemon juice

- Salt and pepper to taste

Instructions:

1. Preheat oven to 375°F (190°C).

2. Season salmon fillets with salt, pepper, and a drizzle of olive oil.

3. Place salmon on a baking sheet lined with parchment paper and bake for 12-15 minutes until cooked through and flaky.

4. In a large bowl, toss together cooked quinoa, mixed salad greens, diced cucumber, and cherry tomatoes.

5. In a small bowl, whisk together olive oil and lemon juice to make the dressing.

6. Divide the salad mixture onto plates and top with baked salmon fillets.

7. Drizzle salad with dressing.

8. Serve immediately and enjoy!

Nutritional Information (per serving):

- Calories: 350

- Protein: 25g

- Carbohydrates: 20g

- Fat: 18g

- Fiber: 4g

4. Veggie Stir-Fry with Tofu

Prep Time: 15 minutes

Cooking Time: 15 minutes

Serving Size: 2

Ingredients:

- 1 block firm tofu, cubed

- 2 cups mixed vegetables (such as bell peppers, broccoli, carrots, snap peas)

- 2 tablespoons low-sodium soy sauce

- 1 tablespoon sesame oil

- 2 cloves garlic, minced

- 1 teaspoon grated ginger

- Cooked brown rice for serving

Instructions:

1. Heat sesame oil in a large skillet or wok over medium heat.

2. Add cubed tofu to the skillet and cook for 5-7 minutes until golden brown and crispy on all sides.

3. Remove tofu from the skillet and set aside.

4. In the same skillet, add mixed vegetables, minced garlic, and grated ginger. Stir-fry for 5-7 minutes until vegetables are tender-crisp.

5. Return tofu to the skillet and toss with vegetables.

6. Drizzle with low-sodium soy sauce and toss to coat evenly.

7. Serve stir-fry over cooked brown rice.

Nutritional Information (per serving):

- Calories: 300

- Protein: 20g

- Carbohydrates: 30g

- Fat: 12g

- Fiber: 8g

5. Quinoa and Black Bean Salad

Prep Time: 15 minutes

Cooking Time: 15 minutes

Serving Size: 4

Ingredients:

- 1 cup cooked quinoa

- 1 cup canned black beans, drained and rinsed

- 1/2 cup corn kernels (fresh or frozen)

- 1/2 cup diced bell peppers

- 1/4 cup chopped cilantro

- 2 tablespoons lime juice

- 1 tablespoon olive oil

- Salt and pepper to taste

Instructions:

1. In a large bowl, combine cooked quinoa, black beans, corn kernels, diced bell peppers, and chopped cilantro.

2. In a small bowl, whisk together lime juice, olive oil, salt, and pepper to make the dressing.

3. Pour the dressing over the quinoa salad and toss to coat evenly.

4. Serve chilled or at room temperature.

Nutritional Information (per serving):

- Calories: 250

- Protein: 10g

- Carbohydrates: 40g

- Fat: 6g

- Fiber: 8g

6. Chicken and Vegetable Soup

Prep Time: 15 minutes

Cooking Time: 30 minutes

Serving Size: 4

Ingredients:

- 2 boneless, skinless chicken breasts, diced

- 4 cups low-sodium chicken broth

- 1 cup diced carrots

- 1 cup diced celery

- 1 cup diced onions

- 2 cloves garlic, minced

- 1 teaspoon dried thyme

- Salt and pepper to taste

- Chopped fresh parsley for garnish

Instructions:

1. In a large pot, bring chicken broth to a simmer over medium heat.

2. Add diced chicken breasts, carrots, celery, onions, minced garlic, and dried thyme to the pot.

3. Season with salt and pepper to taste.

4. Simmer for 20-25 minutes until chicken is cooked through and vegetables are tender.

5. Taste and adjust seasoning if needed.

6. Ladle soup into bowls and garnish with chopped fresh parsley.

7. Serve hot and enjoy!

Nutritional Information (per serving):

- Calories: 200

- Protein: 25g

- Carbohydrates: 15g

- Fat: 4g

- Fiber: 3g

7. Turkey and Vegetable Quinoa Bowl

Prep Time: 15 minutes

Cooking Time: 20 minutes

Serving Size: 2

Ingredients:

- 1 cup cooked quinoa

- 8 ounces lean ground turkey

- 1 cup mixed vegetables (such as bell peppers, zucchini, squash)

- 2 cloves garlic, minced

- 2 tablespoons low-sodium soy sauce

- 1 tablespoon olive oil

- Salt and pepper to taste

Instructions:

1. Heat olive oil in a large skillet over medium heat.

2. Add minced garlic and cook for 1 minute until fragrant.

3. Add ground turkey to the skillet and cook until browned and cooked through, breaking it apart with a spoon.

4. Add mixed vegetables to the skillet and cook for 5-7 minutes until tender.

5. Stir in cooked quinoa and low-sodium soy sauce.

6. Season with salt and pepper to taste.

7. Cook for another 2-3 minutes until everything is heated through.

8. Serve turkey and vegetable quinoa mixture in bowls.

Nutritional Information (per serving):

- Calories: 300

- Protein: 25g

- Carbohydrates: 30g

- Fat: 10g

- Fiber: 6g

8. Baked Cod with Lemon and Herbs

Prep Time: 10 minutes

Cooking Time: 15 minutes

Serving Size: 2

Ingredients:

- 2 cod fillets

- 2 tablespoons olive oil

- 1 tablespoon lemon juice

- 1 teaspoon dried herbs (such as thyme, oregano, or dill)

- Salt and pepper to taste

- Lemon slices for garnish

Instructions:

1. Preheat oven to 400°F (200°C).

2. Place cod fillets on a baking sheet lined with parchment paper.

3. In a small bowl, whisk together olive oil, lemon juice, dried herbs, salt, and pepper.

4. Brush the mixture over the cod fillets, coating them evenly.

5. Place lemon slices on top of the cod fillets.

6. Bake for 12-15 minutes until the fish is opaque and flakes easily with a fork.

7. Serve baked cod with lemon slices.

Nutritional Information (per serving):

- Calories: 200

- Protein: 25g

- Carbohydrates: 2g

- Fat: 10g

- Fiber: 0g

9. Vegetable and Lentil Soup

Prep Time: 15 minutes

Cooking Time: 30 minutes

Serving Size: 4

Ingredients:

- 1 cup dried green lentils, rinsed

- 4 cups vegetable broth

- 1 cup diced carrots

- 1 cup diced celery

- 1 cup diced onions

- 2 cloves garlic, minced

- 1 teaspoon ground cumin

- 1/2 teaspoon paprika

- Salt and pepper to taste

- Chopped fresh parsley for garnish

Instructions:

1. In a large pot, combine dried lentils and vegetable broth.

2. Bring to a boil over medium-high heat, then reduce heat to low and simmer for 15 minutes.

3. Add diced carrots, celery, onions, minced garlic, ground cumin, and paprika to the pot.

4. Season with salt and pepper to taste.

5. Continue to simmer for another 15-20 minutes until lentils and vegetables are tender.

6. Taste and adjust seasoning if needed.

7. Ladle soup into bowls and garnish with chopped fresh parsley.

8. Serve hot and enjoy!

Nutritional Information (per serving):

- Calories: 250

- Protein: 15g

- Carbohydrates: 40g

- Fat: 2g

- Fiber: 15g

10. Mediterranean Chickpea Salad

Prep Time: 15 minutes

Serving Size: 4

Ingredients:

- 1 can (15 ounces) chickpeas, drained and rinsed

- 1 cup diced cucumber

- 1 cup halved cherry tomatoes

- 1/4 cup diced red onion

- 1/4 cup chopped fresh parsley

- 2 tablespoons olive oil

- 1 tablespoon lemon juice

- 1 teaspoon dried oregano

- Salt and pepper to taste

Instructions:

1. In a large bowl, combine chickpeas, diced cucumber, halved cherry tomatoes, diced red onion, and chopped fresh parsley.

2. In a small bowl, whisk together olive oil, lemon juice, dried oregano, salt, and pepper to make the dressing.

3. Pour the dressing over the chickpea salad and toss to coat evenly.

4. Serve chilled or at room temperature.

Nutritional Information (per serving):

- Calories: 200

- Protein: 8g

- Carbohydrates: 25g

- Fat: 8g

- Fiber: 7g

11. Turkey and Spinach Stuffed Peppers

Prep Time: 20 minutes

Cooking Time: 30 minutes

Serving Size: 4

Ingredients:

- 4 bell peppers, halved and seeds removed

- 8 ounces lean ground turkey

- 1 cup cooked quinoa

- 1 cup chopped spinach

- 1/2 cup diced tomatoes

- 1/4 cup diced onions

- 2 cloves garlic, minced

- 1 teaspoon dried Italian herbs

- Salt and pepper to taste

- 1/2 cup shredded low-fat cheese (optional)

Instructions:

1. Preheat oven to 375°F (190°C).

2. Place the halved bell peppers in a baking dish.

3. In a skillet, cook ground turkey over medium heat until browned.

4. Add minced garlic, diced onions, and chopped spinach to the skillet. Cook until the spinach wilts and the onions are translucent.

5. Stir in cooked quinoa, diced tomatoes, dried Italian herbs, salt, and pepper. Cook for an additional 2-3 minutes until well combined.

6. Spoon the turkey and quinoa mixture into each bell pepper half.

7. If desired, sprinkle shredded low-fat cheese on top of each stuffed pepper.

8. Cover the baking dish with aluminum foil and bake for 25-30 minutes until the peppers are tender.

9. Remove the foil and bake for an additional 5 minutes until the cheese is melted and bubbly.

10. Serve hot and enjoy!

Nutritional Information (per serving):

- Calories: 250

- Protein: 20g

- Carbohydrates: 20g

- Fat: 8g

- Fiber: 5g

12. Shrimp and Avocado Salad

Prep Time: 15 minutes

Cooking Time: 5 minutes

Serving Size: 2

Ingredients:

- 8 ounces shrimp, peeled and deveined

- 2 cups mixed salad greens

- 1 avocado, diced

- 1/2 cup cherry tomatoes, halved

- 1/4 cup sliced red onion

- 2 tablespoons olive oil

- 1 tablespoon lemon juice

- Salt and pepper to taste

Instructions:

1. Heat olive oil in a skillet over medium heat.

2. Add shrimp to the skillet and cook for 2-3 minutes per side until pink and cooked through.

3. In a large bowl, toss together mixed salad greens, diced avocado, halved cherry tomatoes, and sliced red onion.

4. In a small bowl, whisk together olive oil and lemon juice to make the dressing.

5. Drizzle salad with dressing and toss to coat evenly.

6. Divide salad onto plates and top with cooked shrimp.

7. Serve immediately and enjoy!

Nutritional Information (per serving):

- Calories: 300

- Protein: 20g

- Carbohydrates: 15g

- Fat: 20g

- Fiber: 8g

13. Chicken and Vegetable Stir-Fry

Prep Time: 15 minutes

Cooking Time: 15 minutes

Serving Size: 2

Ingredients:

- 2 boneless, skinless chicken breasts, thinly sliced

- 2 cups mixed vegetables (such as broccoli, bell peppers, snap peas)

- 2 cloves garlic, minced

- 2 tablespoons low-sodium soy sauce

- 1 tablespoon olive oil

- 1 teaspoon sesame seeds (optional)

- Cooked brown rice for serving

Instructions:

1. Heat olive oil in a large skillet or wok over medium-high heat.

2. Add minced garlic to the skillet and cook for 1 minute until fragrant.

3. Add sliced chicken breasts to the skillet and cook for 5-7 minutes until browned and cooked through.

4. Add mixed vegetables to the skillet and stir-fry for 5-7 minutes until tender-crisp.

5. Drizzle low-sodium soy sauce over the chicken and vegetables. Toss to coat evenly.

6. If desired, sprinkle sesame seeds over the stir-fry.

7. Serve stir-fry over cooked brown rice.

Nutritional Information (per serving):

- Calories: 350

- Protein: 30g

- Carbohydrates: 25g

- Fat: 15g

- Fiber: 6g

14. Caprese Salad with Balsamic Glaze

Prep Time: 10 minutes

Serving Size: 2

Ingredients:

- 2 ripe tomatoes, sliced

- 1 ball fresh mozzarella cheese, sliced

- 1/4 cup fresh basil leaves

- 2 tablespoons balsamic glaze

- Salt and pepper to taste

Instructions:

1. Arrange tomato slices and mozzarella slices alternately on a serving plate.

2. Tuck fresh basil leaves between the tomato and mozzarella slices.

3. Drizzle balsamic glaze over the salad.

4. Season with salt and pepper to taste.

5. Serve immediately and enjoy!

Nutritional Information (per serving):

- Calories: 250

- Protein: 12g

- Carbohydrates: 10g

- Fat: 18g

- Fiber: 2g

15. Turkey and Hummus Wrap

Prep Time: 10 minutes

Serving Size: 1

Ingredients:

- 1 whole grain tortilla

- 3 slices deli turkey breast

- 2 tablespoons hummus

- 1/4 cup mixed salad greens

- 1/4 cup shredded carrots

- 1/4 cup sliced cucumber

Instructions:

1. Lay the whole grain tortilla flat on a clean surface.

2. Spread hummus evenly over the tortilla.

3. Layer slices of deli turkey breast, mixed salad greens, shredded carrots, and sliced cucumber on top.

4. Roll up the tortilla tightly into a wrap.

5. Slice in half if desired and serve.

Nutritional Information (per serving):

- Calories: 300

- Protein: 20g

- Carbohydrates: 25g

- Fat: 12g

- Fiber: 6g

16. Tuna Salad Lettuce Wraps

Prep Time: 10 minutes

Serving Size: 2

Ingredients:

- 1 can (5 ounces) tuna, drained

- 2 tablespoons Greek yogurt

- 1 tablespoon lemon juice

- 1/4 cup diced celery

- 1/4 cup diced red onion

- 1 tablespoon chopped fresh dill

- Salt and pepper to taste

- 4 large lettuce leaves (such as romaine or butter lettuce)

Instructions:

1. In a bowl, combine drained tuna, Greek yogurt, lemon juice, diced celery, diced red onion, and chopped fresh dill.

2. Season with salt and pepper to taste.

3. Mix until well combined.

4. Spoon the tuna salad onto lettuce leaves.

5. Wrap the lettuce leaves around the tuna salad filling.

6. Serve immediately and enjoy!

Nutritional Information (per serving):

- Calories: 150

- Protein: 15g

- Carbohydrates: 5g

- Fat: 6g

- Fiber: 2g

17. Roasted Vegetable Quinoa Bowl

Prep Time: 15 minutes

Cooking Time: 25 minutes

Serving Size: 2

Ingredients:

- 1 cup cooked quinoa

- 2 cups mixed vegetables (such as bell peppers, zucchini, eggplant)

- 2 tablespoons olive oil

- 1 teaspoon dried Italian herbs

- Salt and pepper to taste

- 1/4 cup crumbled feta cheese (optional)

Instructions:

1. Preheat oven to 400°F (200°C).

2. Toss mixed vegetables with olive oil, dried Italian herbs, salt, and pepper on a baking sheet.

3. Roast vegetables in the preheated oven for 20-25 minutes until tender and slightly caramelized.

4. Divide cooked quinoa into bowls.

5. Top with roasted vegetables.

6. If desired, sprinkle crumbled feta cheese over the bowls.

7. Serve hot and enjoy!

Nutritional Information (per serving):

- Calories: 300

- Protein: 10g

- Carbohydrates: 35g

- Fat: 15g

- Fiber: 7g

18. Eggplant and Tomato Pasta

Prep Time: 15 minutes

Cooking Time: 25 minutes

Serving Size: 2

Ingredients:

- 6 ounces whole wheat spaghetti

- 1 small eggplant, diced

- 1 cup cherry tomatoes, halved

- 2 cloves garlic, minced

- 2 tablespoons olive oil

- 1/4 cup chopped fresh basil

- Salt and pepper to taste

- Grated Parmesan cheese for serving (optional)

Instructions:

1. Cook whole wheat spaghetti according to package instructions until al dente. Drain and set aside.

2. Heat olive oil in a large skillet over medium heat.

3. Add diced eggplant to the skillet and cook for 8-10 minutes until softened and lightly browned.

4. Add minced garlic to the skillet and cook for 1 minute until fragrant.

5. Stir in halved cherry tomatoes and cook for another 5 minutes until tomatoes are softened.

6. Toss cooked spaghetti with the eggplant and tomato mixture.

7. Season with salt and pepper to taste.

8. Garnish with chopped fresh basil.

9. If desired, sprinkle grated Parmesan cheese over the pasta.

10. Serve hot and enjoy!

Nutritional Information (per serving):

- Calories: 350

- Protein: 10g

- Carbohydrates: 45g

- Fat: 15g

- Fiber: 8g

19. Chicken and Rice Soup

Prep Time: 15 minutes

Cooking Time: 30 minutes

Serving Size: 4

Ingredients:

- 2 boneless, skinless chicken breasts

- 6 cups low-sodium chicken broth

- 1 cup diced carrots

- 1 cup diced celery

- 1 cup diced onions

- 1 cup cooked brown rice

- 2 cloves garlic, minced

- 1 teaspoon dried thyme

- Salt and pepper to taste

- Chopped fresh parsley for garnish

Instructions:

1. In a large pot, bring chicken broth to a simmer over medium heat.

2. Add chicken breasts, diced carrots, diced celery, diced onions, minced garlic, and dried thyme to the pot.

3. Season with salt and pepper to taste.

4. Simmer for 20-25 minutes until chicken is cooked through and vegetables are tender.

5. Remove chicken breasts from the pot and shred with two forks.

6. Return shredded chicken to the pot.

7. Stir in cooked brown rice.

8. Taste and adjust seasoning if needed.

9. Ladle soup into bowls and garnish with chopped fresh parsley.

10. Serve hot and enjoy!

Nutritional Information (per serving):

- Calories: 250

- Protein: 25g

- Carbohydrates: 20g

- Fat: 8g

- Fiber: 4g

20. Lentil and Vegetable Stew

Prep Time: 15 minutes

Cooking Time: 45 minutes

Serving Size: 4

Ingredients:

- 1 cup dried green lentils, rinsed

- 4 cups vegetable broth

- 1 cup diced carrots

- 1 cup diced celery

- 1 cup diced onions

- 2 cloves garlic, minced

- 1 teaspoon ground cumin

- 1/2 teaspoon smoked paprika

- Salt and pepper to taste

- Chopped fresh cilantro for garnish

Instructions:

1. In a large pot, combine dried lentils and vegetable broth.

2. Bring to a boil over medium-high heat, then reduce heat to low and simmer for 15 minutes.

3. Add diced carrots, celery, onions, minced garlic, ground cumin, smoked paprika, salt, and pepper to the pot.

4. Continue to simmer for another 25-30 minutes until lentils and vegetables are tender.

5. Taste and adjust seasoning if needed.

6. Ladle stew into bowls and garnish with chopped fresh cilantro.

7. Serve hot and enjoy!

Nutritional Information (per serving):

- Calories: 200

- Protein: 15g

- Carbohydrates: 30g

- Fat: 2g

- Fiber: 10g

DINNER RECIPES

1. Grilled Salmon with Lemon-Herb Quinoa

Prep Time: 10 minutes

Cooking Time: 15 minutes

Serving Size: 2

Ingredients:

- 2 salmon fillets

- 1 cup quinoa

- 2 cups water or low-sodium chicken broth

- 1 lemon, sliced

- 2 tablespoons olive oil

- 1 tablespoon chopped fresh parsley

- 1 teaspoon dried dill

- Salt and pepper to taste

Instructions:

1. Preheat grill to medium-high heat.

2. Rinse quinoa under cold water and drain.

3. In a saucepan, bring water or chicken broth to a boil. Add quinoa, cover, and simmer for 15 minutes or until liquid is absorbed and quinoa is tender.

4. Meanwhile, brush salmon fillets with olive oil and season with salt, pepper, and dried dill.

5. Grill salmon fillets for 4-5 minutes per side, or until cooked through and flaky.

6. In a small bowl, toss cooked quinoa with chopped parsley and a squeeze of lemon juice.

7. Serve grilled salmon with lemon slices on top of lemon-herb quinoa.

Nutritional Information (per serving):

- Calories: 400

- Protein: 30g

- Carbohydrates: 30g

- Fat: 18g

- Fiber: 4g

2. Chicken and Vegetable Stir-Fry with Brown Rice

Prep Time: 15 minutes

Cooking Time: 15 minutes

Serving Size: 2

Ingredients:

- 2 boneless, skinless chicken breasts, thinly sliced

- 2 cups mixed vegetables (such as bell peppers, broccoli, snap peas)

- 2 cloves garlic, minced

- 2 tablespoons low-sodium soy sauce

- 1 tablespoon olive oil

- 2 cups cooked brown rice

- Salt and pepper to taste

Instructions:

1. Heat olive oil in a large skillet or wok over medium-high heat.

2. Add minced garlic and cook for 1 minute until fragrant.

3. Add sliced chicken breasts to the skillet and cook for 5-7 minutes until browned and cooked through.

4. Add mixed vegetables to the skillet and stir-fry for 5-7 minutes until tender-crisp.

5. Drizzle low-sodium soy sauce over the chicken and vegetables. Toss to coat evenly.

6. Serve stir-fry over cooked brown rice.

Nutritional Information (per serving):

- Calories: 400

- Protein: 30g

- Carbohydrates: 45g

- Fat: 10g

- Fiber: 6g

3. Turkey Meatballs with Zucchini Noodles

Prep Time: 20 minutes

Cooking Time: 20 minutes

Serving Size: 2

Ingredients:

- 8 ounces lean ground turkey

- 1/4 cup breadcrumbs (gluten-free if desired)

- 1 egg

- 2 cloves garlic, minced

- 1/4 cup grated Parmesan cheese

- 1 teaspoon dried Italian herbs

- Salt and pepper to taste

- 2 medium zucchini

- 1 cup marinara sauce

- Chopped fresh basil for garnish

Instructions:

1. In a bowl, combine ground turkey, breadcrumbs, egg, minced garlic, grated Parmesan cheese, dried Italian herbs, salt, and pepper. Mix until well combined.

2. Roll the mixture into meatballs, about 1 inch in diameter.

3. Heat olive oil in a large skillet over medium heat. Add meatballs and cook for 8-10 minutes, turning occasionally, until browned and cooked through.

4. While the meatballs are cooking, spiralize the zucchini into noodles.

5. Once the meatballs are cooked, remove them from the skillet and set aside.

6. In the same skillet, add marinara sauce and zucchini noodles. Cook for 3-4 minutes until the noodles are tender.

7. Return the meatballs to the skillet and toss to coat with the sauce.

8. Garnish with chopped fresh basil before serving.

Nutritional Information (per serving):

- Calories: 350

- Protein: 25g

- Carbohydrates: 20g

- Fat: 15g

- Fiber: 4g

4. Baked Cod with Roasted Vegetables

Prep Time: 15 minutes

Cooking Time: 20 minutes

Serving Size: 2

Ingredients:

- 2 cod fillets

- 2 cups mixed vegetables (such as bell peppers, zucchini, cherry tomatoes)

- 2 tablespoons olive oil

- 1 teaspoon dried Italian herbs

- Salt and pepper to taste

- Lemon wedges for serving

Instructions:

1. Preheat oven to 400°F (200°C).

2. Toss mixed vegetables with olive oil, dried Italian herbs, salt, and pepper on a baking sheet.

3. Place cod fillets on top of the vegetables.

4. Drizzle a little olive oil over the cod fillets and season with salt and pepper.

5. Bake in the preheated oven for 15-20 minutes until the fish is opaque and flakes easily with a fork, and the vegetables are tender.

6. Serve baked cod with roasted vegetables alongside lemon wedges for squeezing over the fish.

Nutritional Information (per serving):

- Calories: 300

- Protein: 25g

- Carbohydrates: 15g

- Fat: 12g

- Fiber: 5g

5. Vegetable and Tofu Stir-Fry with Rice Noodles

Prep Time: 20 minutes

Cooking Time: 15 minutes

Serving Size: 2

Ingredients:

- 6 ounces rice noodles

- 1 block firm tofu, cubed

- 2 cups mixed vegetables (such as bell peppers, broccoli, carrots)

- 2 cloves garlic, minced

- 2 tablespoons low-sodium soy sauce

- 1 tablespoon sesame oil

- 1 tablespoon rice vinegar

- 1 teaspoon grated ginger

- Salt and pepper to taste

Instructions:

1. Cook rice noodles according to package instructions. Drain and set aside.

2. Heat sesame oil in a large skillet or wok over medium-high heat.

3. Add cubed tofu to the skillet and cook for 5-7 minutes until golden brown and crispy on all sides.

4. Remove tofu from the skillet and set aside.

5. In the same skillet, add mixed vegetables and minced garlic. Stir-fry for 5-7 minutes until vegetables are tender-crisp.

6. Return tofu to the skillet and toss with vegetables.

7. In a small bowl, whisk together low-sodium soy sauce, rice vinegar, grated ginger, salt, and pepper.

8. Pour the sauce over the tofu and vegetables. Toss to coat evenly.

9. Add cooked rice noodles to the skillet and toss to combine.

10. Cook for another 2-3 minutes until everything is heated through.

11. Serve vegetable and tofu stir-fry with rice noodles hot.

Nutritional Information (per serving):

- Calories: 350

- Protein: 15g

- Carbohydrates: 45g

- Fat: 10g

- Fiber: 5g

6. Turkey and Spinach Stuffed Bell Peppers

Prep Time: 20 minutes

Cooking Time: 35 minutes

Serving Size: 4

Ingredients:

- 4 bell peppers, halved and seeds removed

- 8 ounces lean ground turkey

- 1 cup cooked quinoa

- 1 cup chopped spinach

- 1/2 cup diced tomatoes

- 1/4 cup diced onions

- 2 cloves garlic, minced

- 1 teaspoon dried Italian herbs

- Salt and pepper to taste

Instructions:

1. Preheat oven to 375°F (190°C).

2. In a skillet, cook ground turkey over medium heat until browned.

3. Add minced garlic, diced onions, and chopped spinach to the skillet. Cook until the spinach wilts and the onions are translucent.

4. Stir in cooked quinoa, diced tomatoes, dried Italian herbs, salt, and pepper. Cook for an additional 2-3 minutes until well combined.

5. Spoon the turkey and quinoa mixture into each bell pepper half.

6. Place stuffed bell peppers in a baking dish.

7. Cover the baking dish with aluminum foil and bake for 25-30 minutes until the peppers are tender.

8. Remove the foil and bake for an additional 5 minutes until the tops are slightly golden.

9. Serve turkey and spinach stuffed bell peppers hot.

Nutritional Information (per serving):

- Calories: 300

- Protein: 20g

- Carbohydrates: 25g

- Fat: 10g

- Fiber: 5g

7. Grilled Chicken Caesar Salad

Prep Time: 15 minutes

Cooking Time: 15 minutes

Serving Size: 2

Ingredients:

- 2 boneless, skinless chicken breasts

- 4 cups romaine lettuce, chopped

- 1/4 cup grated Parmesan cheese

- 1/2 cup croutons (optional)

- 1/4 cup Caesar dressing

- Salt and pepper to taste

- Lemon wedges for serving

Instructions:

1. Preheat grill to medium-high heat.

2. Season chicken breasts with salt and pepper.

3. Grill chicken for 6-7 minutes per side until cooked through and no longer pink in the center.

4. Slice grilled chicken into thin strips.

5. In a large bowl, toss together chopped romaine lettuce, grated Parmesan cheese, and croutons (if using).

6. Drizzle Caesar dressing over the salad and toss to coat evenly.

7. Divide salad into plates and top with sliced grilled chicken. 8. Serve the grilled chicken Caesar salad with lemon wedges on the side for squeezing over the salad.

Nutritional Information (per serving):

- Calories: 350

- Protein: 30g

- Carbohydrates: 15g

- Fat: 18g

- Fiber: 4g

8. Lentil and Vegetable Curry

Prep Time: 20 minutes

Cooking Time: 30 minutes

Serving Size: 4

Ingredients:

- 1 cup dried green lentils, rinsed

- 4 cups vegetable broth

- 1 cup diced carrots

- 1 cup diced potatoes

- 1 cup diced onions

- 2 cloves garlic, minced

- 1 tablespoon curry powder

- 1 teaspoon ground turmeric

- 1/2 teaspoon ground cumin

- 1/2 teaspoon ground coriander

- 1 can (14 ounces) coconut milk

- Salt and pepper to taste

- Chopped fresh cilantro for garnish

Instructions:

1. In a large pot, combine dried lentils and vegetable broth.

2. Bring to a boil over medium-high heat, then reduce heat to low and simmer for 15 minutes.

3. Add diced carrots, potatoes, onions, minced garlic, curry powder, ground turmeric, ground cumin, and ground coriander to the pot.

4. Simmer for another 15-20 minutes until lentils and vegetables are tender.

5. Stir in coconut milk and simmer for an additional 5 minutes.

6. Taste and adjust seasoning with salt and pepper.

7. Ladle curry into bowls and garnish with chopped fresh cilantro.

8. Serve hot with steamed rice or naan bread.

Nutritional Information (per serving):

- Calories: 350

- Protein: 15g

- Carbohydrates: 45g

- Fat: 12g

- Fiber: 10g

9. Baked Turkey Meatloaf

Prep Time: 15 minutes

Cooking Time: 1 hour

Serving Size: 4

Ingredients:

- 1 pound lean ground turkey

- 1/2 cup breadcrumbs (gluten-free if desired)

- 1/4 cup finely chopped onions

- 1/4 cup grated Parmesan cheese

- 1/4 cup low-sodium ketchup

- 1 egg

- 2 cloves garlic, minced

- 1 teaspoon dried Italian herbs

- Salt and pepper to taste

Instructions:

1. Preheat oven to 375°F (190°C).

2. In a large bowl, combine ground turkey, breadcrumbs, chopped onions, grated Parmesan cheese, ketchup, egg, minced garlic, dried Italian herbs, salt, and pepper.

3. Mix until well combined.

4. Transfer the mixture to a loaf pan and press down evenly.

5. Bake in the preheated oven for 45-60 minutes until cooked through and the top is golden brown.

6. Remove from the oven and let it rest for 5 minutes before slicing.

7. Serve slices of baked turkey meatloaf with your choice of sides, such as mashed potatoes and steamed vegetables.

Nutritional Information (per serving):

- Calories: 250

- Protein: 25g

- Carbohydrates: 15g

- Fat: 10g

- Fiber: 2g

10. Lemon Herb Chicken with Roasted Vegetables

Prep Time: 20 minutes

Cooking Time: 30 minutes

Serving Size: 2

Ingredients:

- 2 boneless, skinless chicken breasts

- 2 cups mixed vegetables (such as bell peppers, carrots, zucchini)

- 2 tablespoons olive oil

- 2 tablespoons lemon juice

- 1 tablespoon chopped fresh parsley

- 1 teaspoon dried thyme

- Salt and pepper to taste

- Lemon wedges for serving

Instructions:

1. Preheat oven to 400°F (200°C).

2. In a small bowl, whisk together olive oil, lemon juice, chopped fresh parsley, dried thyme, salt, and pepper.

3. Place chicken breasts in a baking dish and brush with the lemon herb mixture.

4. Arrange mixed vegetables around the chicken breasts in the baking dish.

5. Drizzle any remaining lemon herb mixture over the vegetables.

6. Bake in the preheated oven for 25-30 minutes until the chicken is cooked through and the vegetables are tender.

7. Serve lemon herb chicken with roasted vegetables hot, with lemon wedges on the side.

Nutritional Information (per serving):

- Calories: 300

- Protein: 30g

- Carbohydrates: 15g

- Fat: 15g

- Fiber: 5g

11. Quinoa Stuffed Bell Peppers

Prep Time: 20 minutes

Cooking Time: 35 minutes

Serving Size: 4

Ingredients:

- 4 large bell peppers, halved and seeds removed

- 1 cup quinoa, rinsed

- 2 cups vegetable broth

- 1 can (15 ounces) black beans, drained and rinsed

- 1 cup corn kernels

- 1 cup diced tomatoes

- 1/2 cup diced onions

- 2 cloves garlic, minced

- 1 teaspoon ground cumin

- 1 teaspoon chili powder

- Salt and pepper to taste

- 1/2 cup shredded cheddar cheese (optional)

- Chopped fresh cilantro for garnish

Instructions:

1. Preheat oven to 375°F (190°C).

2. In a saucepan, bring vegetable broth to a boil. Add quinoa, cover, and simmer for 15-20 minutes until liquid is absorbed and quinoa is tender.

3. In a large bowl, combine cooked quinoa, black beans, corn kernels, diced tomatoes, diced onions, minced garlic, ground cumin, chili powder, salt, and pepper. Mix well.

4. Arrange bell pepper halves in a baking dish.

5. Spoon quinoa mixture into each bell pepper half until filled.

6. If desired, sprinkle shredded cheddar cheese over the stuffed peppers.

7. Cover the baking dish with aluminum foil and bake for 25-30 minutes until the peppers are tender.

8. Remove the foil and bake for an additional 5 minutes until the cheese is melted and bubbly.

9. Garnish with chopped fresh cilantro before serving.

Nutritional Information (per serving):

- Calories: 350

- Protein: 15g

- Carbohydrates: 60g

- Fat: 5g

- Fiber: 12g

12. Lemon Garlic Shrimp Pasta

Prep Time: 15 minutes

Cooking Time: 15 minutes

Serving Size: 2

Ingredients:

- 6 ounces whole wheat spaghetti

- 8 ounces shrimp, peeled and deveined

- 2 tablespoons olive oil

- 4 cloves garlic, minced

- 1 lemon, zest and juice

- 1/4 cup chopped fresh parsley

- Salt and pepper to taste

- Grated Parmesan cheese for serving (optional)

Instructions:

1. Cook whole wheat spaghetti according to package instructions until al dente. Drain and set aside.

2. In a large skillet, heat olive oil over medium heat.

3. Add minced garlic to the skillet and cook for 1 minute until fragrant.

4. Add shrimp to the skillet and cook for 2-3 minutes per side until pink and opaque.

5. Stir in lemon zest and lemon juice.

6. Toss cooked spaghetti with the shrimp mixture.

7. Season with salt and pepper to taste.

8. Garnish with chopped fresh parsley and grated Parmesan cheese if desired.

9. Serve lemon garlic shrimp pasta hot.

Nutritional Information (per serving):

- Calories: 400

- Protein: 25g

- Carbohydrates: 45g

- Fat: 15g

- Fiber: 6g

13. Turkey and Vegetable Skillet

Prep Time: 15 minutes

Cooking Time: 20 minutes

Serving Size: 2

Ingredients:

- 8 ounces lean ground turkey

- 1 cup diced bell peppers

- 1 cup diced zucchini

- 1 cup diced tomatoes

- 1/2 cup diced onions

- 2 cloves garlic, minced

- 1 teaspoon dried Italian herbs

- Salt and pepper to taste

- 1 tablespoon olive oil

- Cooked brown rice for serving

Instructions:

1. Heat olive oil in a large skillet over medium heat.

2. Add diced onions and minced garlic to the skillet. Cook for 2-3 minutes until softened.

3. Add ground turkey to the skillet and cook until browned.

4. Stir in diced bell peppers, diced zucchini, and diced tomatoes.

5. Season with dried Italian herbs, salt, and pepper.

6. Cook for 8-10 minutes until vegetables are tender.

7. Serve turkey and vegetable skillet over cooked brown rice.

Nutritional Information (per serving):

- Calories: 350

- Protein: 25g

- Carbohydrates: 30g

- Fat: 15g

- Fiber: 6g

14. Baked Chicken Parmesan

Prep Time: 20 minutes

Cooking Time: 25 minutes

Serving Size: 2

Ingredients:

- 2 boneless, skinless chicken breasts

- 1/2 cup breadcrumbs (gluten-free if desired)

- 1/4 cup grated Parmesan cheese

- 1 teaspoon dried Italian herbs

- 1/2 cup marinara sauce

- 1/2 cup shredded mozzarella cheese

- Fresh basil leaves for garnish

- Salt and pepper to taste

Instructions:

1. Preheat oven to 400°F (200°C).

2. Season chicken breasts with salt and pepper.

3. In a shallow dish, combine breadcrumbs, grated Parmesan cheese, and dried Italian herbs.

4. Dredge each chicken breast in the breadcrumb mixture, pressing to adhere.

5. Place breaded chicken breasts on a baking sheet lined with parchment paper.

6. Bake in the preheated oven for 15 minutes.

7. Remove from the oven and spoon marinara sauce over each chicken breast.

8. Sprinkle shredded mozzarella cheese over the sauce.

9. Return to the oven and bake for an additional 10 minutes until the cheese is melted and bubbly.

10. Garnish with fresh basil leaves before serving.

Nutritional Information (per serving):

- Calories: 350

- Protein: 30g

- Carbohydrates: 15g

- Fat: 15g

- Fiber: 2g

15. Vegetable and Chickpea Curry

Prep Time: 20 minutes

Cooking Time: 25 minutes

Serving Size: 4

Ingredients:

- 1 tablespoon olive oil

- 1 cup diced onions

- 2 cloves garlic, minced

- 2 teaspoons curry powder

- 1 teaspoon ground cumin

- 1/2 teaspoon ground turmeric

- 1/4 teaspoon cayenne pepper (optional)

- 1 can (14 ounces) diced tomatoes

- 1 can (14 ounces) coconut milk

- 2 cups mixed vegetables (such as bell peppers, carrots, peas)

- 1 can (14 ounces) chickpeas, drained and rinsed

- Salt and pepper to taste

- Chopped fresh cilantro for garnish

Instructions:

1. Heat olive oil in a large skillet over medium heat.

2. Add diced onions to the skillet and cook for 2-3 minutes until softened.

3. Add minced garlic, curry powder, ground cumin, ground turmeric, and cayenne pepper (if using). Cook for 1 minute until fragrant.

4. Stir in diced tomatoes and coconut milk.

5. Add mixed vegetables and chickpeas to the skillet.

6. Bring the mixture to a simmer and cook for 15-20 minutes, stirring occasionally, until the vegetables are tender and the sauce has thickened.

7. Season with salt and pepper to taste.

8. Garnish with chopped fresh cilantro before serving.

9. Serve vegetable and chickpea curry hot with steamed rice or naan bread.

Nutritional Information (per serving):

- Calories: 300

- Protein: 10g

- Carbohydrates: 30g

- Fat: 15g

- Fiber: 8g

16. Baked Salmon with Asparagus

Prep Time: 10 minutes

Cooking Time: 20 minutes

Serving Size: 2

Ingredients:

- 2 salmon fillets

- 1 bunch asparagus, trimmed

- 2 tablespoons olive oil

- 2 cloves garlic, minced

- 1 lemon, sliced

- Salt and pepper to taste

Instructions:

1. Preheat oven to 400°F (200°C).

2. Place salmon fillets on a baking sheet lined with parchment paper.

3. Drizzle olive oil over the salmon fillets and season with minced garlic, salt, and pepper.

4. Arrange trimmed asparagus around the salmon fillets on the baking sheet.

5. Place lemon slices on top of the salmon fillets.

6. Bake in the preheated oven for 15-20 minutes until the salmon is cooked through and flakes easily with a fork, and the asparagus is tender.

7. Serve baked salmon with asparagus hot.

Nutritional Information (per serving):

- Calories: 350

- Protein: 30g

- Carbohydrates: 10g

- Fat: 20g

- Fiber: 5g

17. Turkey Chili

Prep Time: 15 minutes

Cooking Time: 30 minutes

Serving Size: 4

Ingredients:

- 1 tablespoon olive oil

- 1 pound ground turkey

- 1 onion, diced

- 2 cloves garlic, minced

- 1 bell pepper, diced

- 1 can (14 ounces) diced tomatoes

- 1 can (15 ounces) kidney beans, drained and rinsed

- 1 can (15 ounces) black beans, drained and rinsed

- 2 cups low-sodium chicken broth

- 2 tablespoons tomato paste

- 1 tablespoon chili powder

- 1 teaspoon ground cumin

- Salt and pepper to taste

- Chopped fresh cilantro for garnish

- Greek yogurt for serving (optional)

Instructions:

1. Heat olive oil in a large pot over medium heat.

2. Add ground turkey to the pot and cook until browned.

3. Add diced onion, minced garlic, and diced bell pepper to the pot. Cook for 2-3 minutes until softened.

4. Stir in diced tomatoes, kidney beans, black beans, low-sodium chicken broth, tomato paste, chili powder, ground cumin, salt, and pepper.

5. Bring the chili to a simmer and cook for 20-25 minutes, stirring occasionally, until flavors are well combined and chili has thickened.

6. Taste and adjust seasoning if needed.

7. Serve turkey chili hot, garnished with chopped fresh cilantro and a dollop of Greek yogurt if desired.

Nutritional Information (per serving):

- Calories: 300

- Protein: 25g

- Carbohydrates: 30g

- Fat: 10g

- Fiber: 10g

18. Veggie Packed Turkey Meatballs

Prep Time: 20 minutes

Cooking Time: 25 minutes

Serving Size: 4

Ingredients:

- 1 pound lean ground turkey

- 1/2 cup grated zucchini

- 1/2 cup grated carrots

- 1/4 cup diced onions

- 2 cloves garlic, minced

- 1/4 cup breadcrumbs (gluten-free if desired)

- 1 egg

- 1 tablespoon chopped fresh parsley

- 1 teaspoon dried Italian herbs

- Salt and pepper to taste

- Olive oil for cooking

Instructions:

1. Preheat oven to 400°F (200°C). Line a baking sheet with parchment paper.

2. In a large bowl, combine ground turkey, grated zucchini, grated carrots, diced onions, minced garlic, breadcrumbs, egg, chopped fresh parsley, dried Italian herbs, salt, and pepper. Mix until well combined.

3. Shape the mixture into meatballs, about 1 inch in diameter.

4. Place the meatballs on the prepared baking sheet.

5. Drizzle olive oil over the meatballs.

6. Bake in the preheated oven for 20-25 minutes until golden brown and cooked through.

7. Serve veggie-packed turkey meatballs hot with your favorite sauce or over cooked pasta or zucchini noodles.

Nutritional Information (per serving):

- Calories: 250

- Protein: 25g

- Carbohydrates: 10g

- Fat: 12g

- Fiber: 2g

19. Lemon Garlic Roasted Chicken

Prep Time: 10 minutes

Cooking Time: 40 minutes

Serving Size: 2

Ingredients:

- 2 bone-in, skin-on chicken breasts

- 2 tablespoons olive oil

- 2 cloves garlic, minced

- 1 lemon, zest and juice

- 1 tablespoon chopped fresh parsley

- 1 teaspoon dried thyme

- Salt and pepper to taste

Instructions:

1. Preheat oven to 400°F (200°C). Line a baking sheet with parchment paper.

2. Pat dry the chicken breasts with paper towels.

3. In a small bowl, whisk together olive oil, minced garlic, lemon zest, lemon juice, chopped fresh parsley, dried thyme, salt, and pepper.

4. Rub the lemon garlic mixture all over the chicken breasts.

5. Place the chicken breasts on the prepared baking sheet.

6. Roast in the preheated oven for 35-40 minutes until the chicken is cooked through and juices run clear.

7. Remove from the oven and let it rest for 5 minutes before serving.

8. Serve lemon garlic roasted chicken hot with your favorite side dishes, such as roasted vegetables or mashed potatoes.

Nutritional Information (per serving):

- Calories: 350

- Protein: 30g

- Carbohydrates: 5g

- Fat: 20g

- Fiber: 1g

20. Veggie Stir-Fry with Tofu

Prep Time: 15 minutes

Cooking Time: 15 minutes

Serving Size: 2

Ingredients:

- 1 block firm tofu, cubed

- 2 tablespoons low-sodium soy sauce

- 1 tablespoon sesame oil

- 1 tablespoon olive oil

- 2 cloves garlic, minced

- 1 teaspoon grated ginger

- 2 cups mixed vegetables (such as bell peppers, broccoli, carrots)

- Salt and pepper to taste

- Cooked brown rice for serving

Instructions:

1. Press tofu to remove excess moisture. Cut tofu into cubes and place in a bowl.

2. In a separate small bowl, whisk together low-sodium soy sauce, sesame oil, minced garlic, and grated ginger.

3. Pour the soy sauce mixture over the tofu cubes and toss gently to coat.

4. Heat olive oil in a large skillet or wok over medium-high heat.

5. Add marinated tofu cubes to the skillet and cook for 5-7 minutes until golden brown and crispy on all sides. Remove tofu from skillet and set aside.

6. In the same skillet, add mixed vegetables and stir-fry for 5-7 minutes until tender-crisp.

7. Return tofu to the skillet and toss with vegetables. Season with salt and pepper to taste.

8. Serve veggie stir-fry with tofu hot over cooked brown rice.

Nutritional Information (per serving):

- Calories: 300

- Protein: 15g

- Carbohydrates: 25g

- Fat: 15g

- Fiber: 6g

DESSERT RECIPES

Banana Oatmeal Cookies

Prep Time: 10 minutes

Cooking Time: 12 minutes

Serving Size: Makes 12 cookies

Ingredients:

- 2 ripe bananas, mashed

- 1 cup old-fashioned oats

- 1/4 cup almond flour

- 1/4 cup unsweetened applesauce

- 1 teaspoon vanilla extract

- 1/2 teaspoon ground cinnamon

- 1/4 cup dark chocolate chips (optional)

Instructions:

1. Preheat oven to 350°F (175°C). Line a baking sheet with parchment paper.

2. In a mixing bowl, combine mashed bananas, oats, almond flour, applesauce, vanilla extract, and ground cinnamon. Stir until well combined.

3. If desired, fold in dark chocolate chips.

4. Drop spoonfuls of the cookie dough onto the prepared baking sheet, spacing them evenly apart.

5. Flatten each cookie slightly with the back of a spoon.

6. Bake in the preheated oven for 10-12 minutes until the cookies are golden brown.

7. Remove from the oven and let them cool on the baking sheet for 5 minutes before transferring to a wire rack to cool completely.

Nutritional Information (per serving, 1 cookie):

- Calories: 70

- Protein: 1.5g

- Carbohydrates: 12g

- Fat: 2g

- Fiber: 1.5g

Berry Chia Seed Pudding

Prep Time: 5 minutes (plus chilling time)

Cooking Time: 0 minutes

Serving Size: Makes 2 servings

Ingredients:

- 1 cup unsweetened almond milk

- 1/4 cup chia seeds

- 1 tablespoon maple syrup or honey

- 1/2 teaspoon vanilla extract

- 1/2 cup mixed berries (such as strawberries, blueberries, raspberries)

Instructions:

1. In a bowl, whisk together almond milk, chia seeds, maple syrup or honey, and vanilla extract.

2. Let the mixture sit for 5 minutes, then whisk again to prevent clumping.

3. Cover the bowl and refrigerate for at least 2 hours or overnight, until the pudding thickens.

4. Once the pudding has thickened, stir well to ensure an even consistency.

5. Divide the pudding into serving glasses or bowls.

6. Top with mixed berries.

7. Serve chilled.

Nutritional Information (per serving):

- Calories: 150

- Protein: 4g

- Carbohydrates: 18g

- Fat: 7g

- Fiber: 9g

Baked Apples with Cinnamon

Prep Time: 10 minutes

Cooking Time: 30 minutes

Serving Size: Makes 2 servings

Ingredients:

- 2 large apples (such as Granny Smith or Honeycrisp)

- 1 tablespoon lemon juice

- 1 tablespoon honey or maple syrup

- 1 teaspoon ground cinnamon

Instructions:

1. Preheat oven to 375°F (190°C).

2. Core the apples and slice them into thin rounds.

3. Toss the apple slices with lemon juice to prevent browning.

4. Arrange the apple slices in a baking dish.

5. Drizzle honey or maple syrup over the apple slices.

6. Sprinkle ground cinnamon evenly over the apples.

7. Cover the baking dish with aluminum foil and bake for 20 minutes.

8. Remove the foil and bake for an additional 10 minutes until the apples are tender.

9. Serve baked apples warm, optionally with a dollop of yogurt or a sprinkle of granola.

Nutritional Information (per serving):

- Calories: 120

- Protein: 1g

- Carbohydrates: 30g

- Fat: 0.5g

- Fiber: 5g

Greek Yogurt Parfait with Berries and Almonds

Prep Time: 5 minutes

Assembly Time: 5 minutes

Serving Size: Makes 1 serving

Ingredients:

- 1/2 cup plain Greek yogurt

- 1/4 cup mixed berries (such as strawberries, blueberries, raspberries)

- 1 tablespoon sliced almonds

- 1 teaspoon honey (optional)

Instructions:

1. In a serving glass or bowl, layer plain Greek yogurt, mixed berries, and sliced almonds.

2. Drizzle honey over the top if desired.

3. Serve immediately.

Nutritional Information (per serving):

- Calories: 200

- Protein: 15g

- Carbohydrates: 15g

- Fat: 10g

- Fiber: 3g

Peanut Butter Banana Smoothie

Prep Time: 5 minutes

Blending Time: 2 minutes

Serving Size: Makes 1 serving

Ingredients:

- 1 ripe banana

- 1 tablespoon natural peanut butter

- 1/2 cup plain Greek yogurt

- 1/2 cup unsweetened almond milk

- 1/2 teaspoon ground cinnamon

- 1/2 cup ice cubes

Instructions:

1. In a blender, combine ripe banana, natural peanut butter, plain Greek yogurt, unsweetened almond milk, ground cinnamon, and ice cubes.

2. Blend until smooth and creamy.

3. Pour the smoothie into a glass.

4. Serve immediately.

Nutritional Information (per serving):

- Calories: 300

- Protein: 20g

- Carbohydrates: 30g

- Fat: 12g

- Fiber: 5g

Baked Pears with Honey and Cinnamon

Prep Time: 10 minutes

Cooking Time: 25 minutes

Serving Size: Makes 2 servings

Ingredients:

- 2 ripe pears
- 1 tablespoon honey
- 1/2 teaspoon ground cinnamon
- 1/4 teaspoon ground nutmeg

Instructions:

1. Preheat oven to 375°F (190°C).
2. Slice pears in half lengthwise and remove the cores.
3. Place pear halves cut-side up in a baking dish.
4. Drizzle honey over the pear halves.
5. Sprinkle ground cinnamon and ground nutmeg evenly over the pears.
6. Cover the baking dish with aluminum foil and bake for 20 minutes.
7. Remove the foil and bake for an additional 5 minutes until the pears are tender.
8. Serve baked pears warm.

Nutritional Information (per serving):

- Calories: 120
- Protein: 1g

- Carbohydrates: 30g

- Fat: 0.5g

- Fiber: 5g

Chia Seed Pudding with Mango

Prep Time: 5 minutes (plus chilling time)

Cooking Time: 0 minutes

Serving Size: Makes 2 servings

Ingredients:

- 1 cup unsweetened coconut milk

- 1/4 cup chia seeds

- 1 tablespoon honey or maple syrup

- 1/2 teaspoon vanilla extract

- 1 ripe mango, diced

Instructions:

1. In a mixing bowl, combine unsweetened coconut milk, chia seeds, honey or maple syrup, and vanilla extract.

2. Whisk the mixture until well combined.

3. Cover the bowl and refrigerate for at least 2 hours or overnight, allowing the chia seeds to absorb the liquid and thicken.

4. Once the pudding has reached a thick consistency, give it a good stir to distribute the chia seeds evenly.

5. To serve, spoon the chia seed pudding into serving glasses or bowls.

6. Top with diced mango.

7. Enjoy chilled.

Nutritional Information (per serving):

- Calories: 200

- Protein: 4g

- Carbohydrates: 25g

- Fat: 10g

- Fiber: 9g

Baked Blueberry Oatmeal Cups

Prep Time: 10 minutes

Cooking Time: 25 minutes

Serving Size: Makes 6 oatmeal cups

Ingredients:

- 1 cup old-fashioned oats

- 1/4 cup almond flour

- 1 teaspoon baking powder

- 1/2 teaspoon ground cinnamon

- Pinch of salt

- 1/2 cup unsweetened applesauce

- 1/4 cup maple syrup

- 1/4 cup unsweetened almond milk

- 1 egg

- 1 teaspoon vanilla extract

- 1/2 cup fresh blueberries

Instructions:

1. Preheat oven to 350°F (175°C). Grease a muffin tin or line with paper liners.

2. In a mixing bowl, combine old-fashioned oats, almond flour, baking powder, ground cinnamon, and a pinch of salt.

3. In another bowl, whisk together unsweetened applesauce, maple syrup, unsweetened almond milk, egg, and vanilla extract.

4. Pour the wet ingredients into the dry ingredients and stir until well combined.

5. Gently fold in fresh blueberries.

6. Divide the mixture evenly among the muffin cups.

7. Bake in the preheated oven for 20-25 minutes until the tops are golden brown and a toothpick inserted into the center comes out clean.

8. Allow the oatmeal cups to cool slightly before removing them from the muffin tin.

9. Serve warm or at room temperature.

Nutritional Information (per oatmeal cup):

- Calories: 120

- Protein: 4g

- Carbohydrates: 20g

- Fat: 3g

- Fiber: 2g

Coconut Mango Smoothie Bowl

Prep Time: 5 minutes

Blending Time: 2 minutes

Serving Size: Makes 1 serving

Ingredients:

- 1 ripe mango, peeled and diced

- 1/2 cup unsweetened coconut milk

- 1/2 cup plain Greek yogurt

- 1 tablespoon honey (optional)

- 1/4 cup granola

- 1 tablespoon shredded coconut

- Fresh mint leaves for garnish

Instructions:

1. In a blender, combine diced mango, unsweetened coconut milk, plain Greek yogurt, and honey (if using).

2. Blend until smooth and creamy.

3. Pour the smoothie into a bowl.

4. Top with granola and shredded coconut.

5. Garnish with fresh mint leaves.

6. Serve immediately.

Nutritional Information (per serving):

- Calories: 300

- Protein: 10g

- Carbohydrates: 45g

- Fat: 10g

- Fiber: 6g

Frozen Banana Bites

Prep Time: 10 minutes

Freezing Time: 2 hours

Serving Size: Makes 12 banana bites

Ingredients:

- 2 ripe bananas

- 1/4 cup natural peanut butter

- 1/4 cup dark chocolate chips

- 1 teaspoon coconut oil

- Optional toppings: chopped nuts, shredded coconut

Instructions:

1. Peel the bananas and cut them into 1-inch thick slices.

2. Spread a small amount of peanut butter on top of each banana slice.

3. Place the banana slices on a parchment-lined baking sheet.

4. In a microwave-safe bowl, combine dark chocolate chips and coconut oil.

5. Microwave in 30-second intervals, stirring in between, until the chocolate is melted and smooth.

6. Using a fork, dip each peanut butter-coated banana slice into the melted chocolate, coating it halfway.

7. Place the chocolate-coated banana slices back on the parchment-lined baking sheet.

8. Optional: sprinkle chopped nuts or shredded coconut on top of the chocolate-coated banana slices.

9. Freeze the banana bites for at least 2 hours until the chocolate is set.

10. Once frozen, transfer the banana bites to an airtight container and store them in the freezer.

11. Serve frozen banana bites straight from the freezer as a refreshing dessert or snack.

Nutritional Information (per banana bite):

- Calories: 70

- Protein: 2g

- Carbohydrates: 10g

- Fat: 3.5g

- Fiber: 1.5g

LONG-TERM MANAGEMENT AND MAINTENANCE

Living with acid reflux and GERD requires ongoing management and maintenance to ensure symptom relief and overall well-being. While initial dietary changes and lifestyle adjustments may provide relief, long-term management involves consistent monitoring, making necessary adjustments, and seeking professional guidance when needed.

1. Monitoring Symptoms and Progress

Monitoring symptoms and tracking progress are essential aspects of long-term management for acid reflux and GERD. By keeping a symptom diary, individuals can identify triggers, patterns, and trends that may exacerbate or alleviate their symptoms. This diary should include details such as the timing and severity of symptoms, dietary intake, stress levels, sleep quality, and any other relevant factors.

Regularly assessing symptoms allows individuals to evaluate the effectiveness of their current management strategies and make informed decisions about potential adjustments. For instance, if certain foods consistently trigger symptoms, they can be eliminated or limited from the diet. Likewise, if lifestyle factors such as stress or lack of exercise contribute to symptom flare-ups, strategies for managing these factors can be implemented.

Tracking progress over time enables individuals to observe improvements, identify areas of concern, and make necessary modifications to their management plan. It also provides valuable information for healthcare providers, facilitating more personalized and effective treatment recommendations.

2. Adjusting Your Diet as Needed

Diet plays a crucial role in managing acid reflux and GERD, and dietary adjustments may need to be modified over time based on individual symptoms and tolerance levels. While certain foods are commonly associated with triggering symptoms, the specific triggers can vary from person to person. Therefore, it's essential to pay attention to how different foods affect symptoms and adjust the diet accordingly.

Some general dietary recommendations for managing acid reflux and GERD include:

- Avoiding trigger foods such as spicy, acidic, fatty, or fried foods

- Limiting or avoiding caffeine, alcohol, carbonated beverages, and chocolate

- Eating smaller, more frequent meals to prevent overeating and reduce pressure on the stomach

- Avoiding lying down or going to bed immediately after eating

- Elevating the head of the bed to prevent acid reflux during sleep

In addition to avoiding trigger foods, incorporating more reflux-friendly foods into the diet can help alleviate symptoms and promote digestive health. These include:

- Non-citrus fruits such as bananas, apples, and melons

- Vegetables such as broccoli, carrots, and green beans

- Lean proteins such as poultry, fish, and tofu

- Whole grains such as oats, brown rice, and quinoa

- Low-fat dairy products such as yogurt and skim milk

However, individual tolerance to these foods may vary, so it's essential to pay attention to how the body responds and make adjustments as needed. Keeping a food diary can be helpful in identifying problematic foods and guiding dietary modifications.

In some cases, working with a registered dietitian or nutritionist who specializes in digestive health can provide personalized dietary guidance and support. These professionals can help individuals develop a balanced and sustainable eating plan that meets their nutritional needs while minimizing symptoms of acid reflux and GERD.

3. Incorporating Exercise and Stress Management

In addition to dietary modifications, incorporating regular exercise and stress management techniques can play a crucial role in long-term management of acid reflux and GERD. Exercise helps promote overall digestive health by aiding in weight management, improving gastrointestinal motility, and reducing stress levels.

Engaging in moderate-intensity activities such as walking, cycling, swimming, or yoga for at least 30 minutes most days of the week can help alleviate symptoms and improve overall well-being. However, it's essential to choose activities that are comfortable and enjoyable, as strenuous exercise or activities that involve bending or straining may exacerbate symptoms.

Stress is a common trigger for acid reflux and GERD symptoms, so implementing stress management techniques can be beneficial for symptom relief. These may include:

- Practicing relaxation techniques such as deep breathing, meditation, or progressive muscle relaxation

- Engaging in hobbies or activities that promote relaxation and enjoyment

- Prioritizing sleep and establishing a regular sleep schedule

- Seeking support from friends, family, or a mental health professional if stress levels are overwhelming

By incorporating regular exercise and stress management techniques into daily life, individuals can reduce the frequency and severity of acid reflux and GERD symptoms while improving overall quality of life.

4. Seeking Professional Help When Necessary

While dietary and lifestyle modifications are often effective for managing acid reflux and GERD, some individuals may require additional support from healthcare professionals. If symptoms persist despite adherence to recommended strategies or if new or worsening symptoms develop, it's essential to seek medical evaluation and guidance.

Healthcare providers such as primary care physicians, gastroenterologists, or registered dietitians can offer personalized assessment and treatment recommendations based on individual needs and circumstances. This may involve:

- Conducting a thorough medical history and physical examination to identify potential underlying causes or contributing factors

- Ordering diagnostic tests such as endoscopy, pH monitoring, or imaging studies to evaluate the severity of acid reflux and GERD and rule out other conditions

- Prescribing medications such as proton pump inhibitors (PPIs), H2 blockers, or antacids to reduce acid production and relieve symptoms

- Referring to other specialists such as allergists, otolaryngologists, or pulmonologists for further evaluation and management of related conditions

- Providing education and counseling on lifestyle modifications, dietary strategies, and stress management techniques

In some cases, surgical intervention may be recommended for individuals who do not respond to conservative treatments or who have complications such as Barrett's esophagus or severe esophageal damage. Surgical options may include fundoplication, LINX device placement, or endoscopic procedures.

Overall, seeking timely and appropriate medical care is essential for effectively managing acid reflux and GERD and preventing long-term complications. Collaboration between individuals, healthcare providers, and other

30-DAY MEAL PLAN

Day 1:

- Breakfast: Greek Yogurt Parfait with Berries and Granola
- Lunch: Quinoa Salad with Roasted Vegetables
- Dinner: Grilled Salmon with Asparagus
- Dessert: Baked Pears with Honey and Cinnamon

Day 2:

- Breakfast: Spinach and Feta Omelette
- Lunch: Chickpea Salad with Cucumber and Tomato
- Dinner: Chicken and Vegetable Curry with Brown Rice
- Dessert: Berry Chia Seed Pudding

Day 3:

- Breakfast: Overnight Oats with Chia Seeds and Berries
- Lunch: Mediterranean Quinoa Bowl
- Dinner: Spaghetti Squash with Turkey Meatballs
- Dessert: Greek Yogurt Parfait with Berries and Almonds

Day 4:

- Breakfast: Banana Nut Muffins

- Lunch: Spinach and Strawberry Salad with Balsamic Dressing

- Dinner: Baked Chicken Parmesan with Zucchini Noodles

- Dessert: Baked Apples with Cinnamon

Day 5:

- Breakfast: Veggie Omelette with Whole Wheat Toast

- Lunch: Asian-Inspired Tofu Lettuce Wraps

- Dinner: Stuffed Bell Peppers with Quinoa and Black Beans

- Dessert: Chia Seed Pudding with Mango

Day 6:

- Breakfast: Blueberry Banana Smoothie Bowl

- Lunch: Zucchini Noodles with Pesto and Cherry Tomatoes

- Dinner: Lemon Garlic Shrimp with Quinoa Pilaf

- Dessert: Coconut Mango Smoothie Bowl

Day 7:

- Breakfast: Scrambled Tofu Breakfast Burrito

- Lunch: Greek Chicken Pita Pocket with Tzatziki Sauce

- Dinner: Ratatouille with Garlic Bread

- Dessert: Frozen Banana Bites

Day 8:

- Breakfast: Peanut Butter Banana Overnight Oats

- Lunch: Salmon Caesar Salad with Homemade Dressing

- Dinner: Beef and Broccoli Stir-Fry with Rice Noodles

- Dessert: Baked Blueberry Oatmeal Cups

Day 9:

- Breakfast: Quinoa Breakfast Bowl with Almond Milk and Fruit

- Lunch: Veggie Wrap with Hummus and Roasted Peppers

- Dinner: Eggplant Parmesan with Whole Wheat Pasta

- Dessert: Banana Oatmeal Cookies

Day 10:

- Breakfast: Banana Oatmeal Pancakes

- Lunch: Tomato Basil Soup with Grilled Cheese Sandwich

- Dinner: Thai Coconut Curry with Tofu and Vegetables

- Dessert: Greek Yogurt Parfait with Berries and Almonds

Day 11:

- Breakfast: Veggie Breakfast Casserole with Sweet Potatoes

- Lunch: Quinoa and Black Bean Stuffed Bell Peppers

- Dinner: Black Bean and Sweet Potato Enchiladas

- Dessert: Baked Pears with Honey and Cinnamon

Day 12:

- Breakfast: Chia Seed Pudding with Mango and Coconut

- Lunch: Lentil Shepherd's Pie with Mashed Cauliflower

- Dinner: Mediterranean Baked Chicken with Greek Salad

- Dessert: Berry Chia Seed Pudding

Day 13:

- Breakfast: Baked Eggs in Avocado

- Lunch: Quinoa Stuffed Portobello Mushrooms

- Dinner: Veggie Packed Turkey Meatballs with Marinara Sauce

- Dessert: Baked Apples with Cinnamon

Day 14:

- Breakfast: Breakfast Tacos with Black Beans and Salsa

- Lunch: Caprese Salad with Balsamic Glaze

- Dinner: Baked Cod with Roasted Vegetables

- Dessert: Peanut Butter Banana Smoothie

Day 15:

- Breakfast: Sweet Potato Hash with Eggs

- Lunch: Lentil Soup with Spinach and Carrots

- Dinner: Mediterranean Quinoa Bowl

- Dessert: Coconut Mango Smoothie Bowl

Day 16:

- Breakfast: Breakfast Quinoa with Almond Butter and Apples

- Lunch: Turkey and Hummus Wrap

- Dinner: Teriyaki Tofu Stir-Fry with Vegetables

- Dessert: Greek Yogurt Parfait with Berries and Almonds

Day 17:

- Breakfast: Apple Cinnamon Baked Oatmeal

- Lunch: Veggie Stir-Fry with Tofu

- Dinner: Mushroom and Spinach Risotto

- Dessert: Chia Seed Pudding with Mango

Day 18:

- Breakfast: Greek Yogurt with Honey and Mixed Berries

- Lunch: Black Bean Quesadilla with Salsa and Guacamole

- Dinner: Thai Coconut Curry with Tofu and Vegetables

- Dessert: Baked Blueberry Oatmeal Cups

Day 19:

- Breakfast: Breakfast Smoothie with Spinach, Mango, and Banana

- Lunch: Chicken and Vegetable Stir-Fry with Brown Rice

- Dinner: Beef and Broccoli Stir-Fry with Rice Noodles

- Dessert: Banana Oatmeal Cookies

Day 20:

- Breakfast: Avocado Toast with Poached Eggs

- Lunch: Greek Salad with Grilled Shrimp

- Dinner: Veggie Packed Turkey Meatballs with Marinara Sauce

- Dessert: Frozen Banana Bites

Day 21:

- Breakfast: Spinach and Feta Omelette

- Lunch: Lentil Shepherd's Pie with Mashed Cauliflower

- Dinner: Grilled Salmon with Asparagus

- Dessert: Baked Apples with Cinnamon

Day 22:

- Breakfast: Overnight Oats with Chia Seeds and Berries

- Lunch: Veggie Wrap with Hummus and Roasted Peppers

- Dinner: Chicken and Vegetable Curry with Brown Rice

- Dessert: Berry Chia Seed Pudding

Day 23:

- Breakfast: Banana Nut Muffins

- Lunch: Quinoa and Black Bean Stuffed Bell Peppers

- Dinner: Spaghetti Squash with Turkey Meatballs

- Dessert: Greek Yogurt Parfait with Berries and Almonds

Day 24:

- Breakfast: Veggie Omelette with Whole Wheat Toast

- Lunch: Tomato Basil Soup with Grilled Cheese Sandwich

- Dinner: Stuffed Bell Peppers with Quinoa and Black Beans

- Dessert: Chia Seed Pudding with Mango

Day 25:

- Breakfast: Blueberry Banana Smoothie Bowl

- Lunch: Asian-Inspired Tofu Lettuce Wraps

- Dinner: Lemon Garlic Shrimp with Quinoa Pilaf

- Dessert: Coconut Mango Smoothie Bowl

Day 26:

- Breakfast: Scrambled Tofu Breakfast Burrito

- Lunch: Greek Chicken Pita Pocket with Tzatziki Sauce

- Dinner: Ratatouille with Garlic Bread

- Dessert: Frozen Banana Bites

Day 27:

- Breakfast: Peanut Butter Banana Overnight Oats

- Lunch: Salmon Caesar Salad with Homemade Dressing

- Dinner: Beef and Broccoli Stir-Fry with Rice Noodles

- Dessert: Baked Blueberry Oatmeal Cups

Day 28:

- Breakfast: Quinoa Breakfast Bowl with Almond Milk and Fruit

- Lunch: Spinach and Strawberry Salad with Balsamic Dressing

- Dinner: Baked Chicken Parmesan with Zucchini Noodles

- Dessert: Baked Apples with Cinnamon

Day 29:

- Breakfast: Banana Oatmeal Pancakes

- Lunch: Mediterranean Quinoa Bowl

- Dinner: Black Bean and Sweet Potato Enchiladas

- Dessert: Banana Oatmeal Cookies

Day 30:

- Breakfast: Veggie Breakfast Casserole with Sweet Potatoes

- Lunch: Caprese Salad with Balsamic Glaze

- Dinner: Baked Cod with Roasted Vegetables

- Dessert: Peanut Butter Banana Smoothie

CONCLUSION

As we draw to a close with the "Acid Reflux and GERD Diet Cookbook for Beginners," it's evident that managing these conditions needn't be daunting or limiting. Throughout this cookbook, we've explored an array of delicious and healthful recipes crafted to alleviate symptoms, bolster digestive health, and enhance overall well-being.

From enticing breakfast choices like avocado toast with poached eggs to hearty dinner selections like grilled salmon with asparagus, each recipe has been meticulously chosen with the principles of an acid reflux and GERD-friendly diet in mind. We've embraced whole foods, lean proteins, and an abundance of fruits and vegetables while minimizing trigger foods that can exacerbate symptoms.

However, beyond merely providing recipes, this cookbook serves as an exhaustive guide for beginners navigating the challenges of acid reflux and GERD. We've delved into the fundamentals of these conditions, examining their causes, symptoms, and potential complications. By grasping the underlying factors at play, readers can make more informed decisions about their dietary and lifestyle choices.

Throughout the book, we've stressed the importance of listening to your body and observing how different foods and behaviors affect your symptoms. Maintaining a food diary, tracking progress, and seeking professional advice when necessary are critical components of long-term management and maintenance.

Furthermore, we've emphasized the significance of integrating lifestyle adjustments such as regular exercise and stress management techniques into your daily routine. By addressing these aspects, individuals can not only alleviate symptoms but also enhance their overall quality of life.

It's essential to remember that managing acid reflux and GERD is not a one-size-fits-all endeavor. What works for one person may not work for another, and it may take some experimentation to discover the optimal combination of dietary and lifestyle strategies that suit your individual needs.

However, with patience, perseverance, and the support of resources like this cookbook, it's possible to find relief and take charge of your digestive health. By adopting a balanced and sustainable approach to eating and living, you can savor delicious meals without sacrificing flavor or satisfaction.

Ultimately, the "Acid Reflux and GERD Diet Cookbook for Beginners" is more than just a collection of recipes—it's a guidebook to improved health and well-being. Whether you're embarking on your journey or seeking new ways to manage your symptoms, let this cookbook be your companion as you chart a course to digestive wellness.

So here's to good health, enjoyable eating, and a future liberated from the discomfort of acid reflux and GERD. May these recipes nourish not only your body but also your spirit, bringing joy and vitality to every meal. Here's to a life filled with flavor, balance, and vibrant health!

9 798320 229065